HS WARRIOR

Congratulations Roberta

Pen

©2016

Stay strong Warrior Pen

ISBN-13: 978-153137829
ISBN-10: 1535137827

The Robber appears in the anthology of HS patient stories, I Will Not Hide with the permission and gratitude of the author.

Cover created by Ron Bercume
www.hsawareness.org
www.hssupport.org

Also visit
www.penspen.wix.com/hswarrior
www.penspen.wix.com/neros-fiddle
www.penspen.wix.com/eightonablade

This book is cat-approved.

This book is for all who suffer from
Hidradenitis Suppurativa.
We are all Warriors.
We are all victorious.

Acknowledgements

I would like to gratefully acknowledge the PenTwin. She has been with me every step of the way through all of my flare-ups and surgeries. Most importantly, she was with me during this latest test of endurance. She is the one person who called me every day to see how I was doing. No matter how much I grumbled, whined or cried in her ear, she steadfastly offered me moral support and encouraged me to hold on if for just one more day. Even during those times when I took out my frustration on her, she was still there for me. That is the definition of a real friend. I would not have survived without her.

And my kitty cat, Clairee, who has also been with me throughout the whole ordeal. At the age of sixteen years, she is still my sunshine and offers unconditional love and gratitude.

And, finally, my family, without whom my creativity would not be possible.

Foreword

Hidradenitis Suppurativa. HS.

It just sounds like a big name for a disease. As you will read in this book, it is much more.

My best friend, Pen, suffers from HS – and I mean SUFFERS, with all caps entirely necessary. We talk every day on the phone and have for years. I was there when her latest flare-up began, and I've heard and felt the agony she's gone through every single day since.

I hear it in her voice. She sounds pained some days – excruciatingly so much of the time. Other days, she sounds physically and emotionally completely drained. Sometimes, I can tell she doesn't even have the energy to talk.

Once in a while, she sounds like her old self on the phone. That makes me happy. But those times are few and far between.

I hate HS.

But HS needs to be in the spotlight – so that the pursuit of a cure also is in the spotlight of the medical community.

I want my friend back. I want HS gone. Read this book, share it, and do something to help. If we all help, HS can lose its power over its victims and their loved ones.

You don't want to know about HS. But you *need* to know. And we all need to band together and make HS history.

Penny Weaver
Mattoon, Illinois

HS Warrior

Table of Contents

Preface

This is not a happy book: There is nothing happy about Hidradenitis Suppurativa.

It is a book about endurance: surviving long days and even longer nights, tolerating the misconceptions and degrading attitudes of those who choose not to understand what HS is; dealing with the lack of compassion from medical personnel and family alike.

It is a book about the journey I have traveled in my quest to overcome this debilitating illness.

It is a lifelong quest. Once you have Hidradenitis Suppurativa, you have it for life. There is currently no cure.

It is a book about the debilitating and devastating effects of HS. Though this book is about my personal experience, the essays contained herein are likely echoes of what many others go through.

Fair warning: Google "Hidradenitis Suppurativa" at your own risk. The images are graphic and disturbing to see.

The actual suffering this illness thrusts upon its victims is much more disturbing than those images project.

I haven't held anything back. The writing is forthright and raw. It simply is not possible to "prettify" Hidradenitis Suppurativa.

Regardless of how raw and forthright it is, overall, this book is about hope: the hope of survival, the hope of raising awareness, the hope of there one day being a cure.

Hope gives me the strength to survive another day.

I can only hope others cling to their hope to survive another day.

Progress of Hidradenitis Suppurativa

When I was in my twenties, I suffered from Hidradenitis Suppurativa. This was back in the 1980s. It was not diagnosed as HS then.

At that time, boils formed, some along my groin, some along my "apron" – the fat that overhangs the labia area. Fortunately, these boils would burst, drain and go away. More would return, usually in different areas, but it was the same: burst, drain, go away.

I was told these were the result of "clogged hair follicles." And they were nothing to worry about.

One doctor, I think, had some fetish about lancing things. She lanced one of them in her office, painfully so, and squeezed it to drain it. It left a scar, but I've never been worried about scars.

On occasion a boil would form directly on my tailbone. This one would get huge. It would be there for days, get painful and, when it finally burst, it drained a large amount. But this, too, would leave only to return on occasion.

I also recall getting some of those boil-like abscesses in my armpits. I noticed very quickly that these occurred mostly when I shaved my armpits. So, I stopped doing that.

3

They still popped up on occasion, but since I stopped using underarm deodorant, I haven't had any more in that location.

In 2008, I told my primary care physician at that time that I was "growing a tail." Several bumps were formed along my tailbone and along the right side of my buttocks. She referred me to a surgeon: a gastrointestinal surgeon.

This surgeon diagnosed it as a pilonidal cyst. With fistula, no less. Seriously? That has to be the most obscene medical term I've ever heard. Of course, he was referring to the "tunnels" which form with HS. In 2008, HS was an unknown.

This first surgery was horrible. I left the hospital with a hole in my backside huge enough to put a fist into. I know because I saw the reflection of it in a mirror. The fist-sized hole provided a fist-sized pain as well. Even after two months off from work, it was still painful to sit when I returned to my job.

The surgeon, as well as my primary care doctor at that time, refused to give me antibiotics. Had I been aware of the risks of staph or MRSA infections, I would have demanded antibiotics. I trusted them because they are doctors and doctors are supposed to know best about these things.

I'm rethinking that trust.

By the second flare-up in 2012, I learned the proper name: Hidradenitis Suppurativa. This surgeon performed a better job. The surgical wounds were not nearly as invasive or painful. But the surgeon herself was the coldest fish I'd ever met.

Now in 2016 with the worst flare-up I've ever had, I can't get surgery without winning the lottery.

I noticed the four-year pattern. It seems my HS can only tolerate prolonged sitting for a period of four years.

Although prolonged sitting is not one of the "causes" attributed to HS, no one really knows for sure. I can state that the first surgeon reported my prolonged sitting as the cause for the pilonidal cyst. I know because his office filed for Worker's Compensation for me (for a fee, of course).

Logically, it stands to reason – at least to me – that prolonged sitting would also be a contributor to HS. But what do I know? I'm not a doctor. But since they don't know what causes it anyway, prolonged sitting should at least be considered.

Oh, but that would make those sit-down jobs responsible, wouldn't it? HS patients could claim Worker's Compensation, couldn't they? And big business doesn't want that.

Be that as it may, consider the progression of HS since the 1980s. From the completely unknown to fistula to it not being recognized as a debilitating illness, even though at least a few more doctors know about it.

I suppose the fact that HS is becoming a more common diagnosis, that can be considered progress. More people are aware of HS. Not enough to foster compassion or to receive any assistance. But achieving that point takes time and vigilance. And a lot of hard work by a lot of people. Including the surgeons who understand HS and treat it.

Maybe in the next four years, by the time my next flare-up is due – provided I survive this one – maybe there will be medication or treatment or a combination of the two to prevent the flare-up. Or to reduce it without surgery.

One can only hope the "progress" of HS progresses that quickly.

The Robber

Like a thief in the night, Hidradenitis Suppurative catches a person unaware. One day things are fine. The next day, these mysterious lumps with nasty, smelly drainage rob you of the person you are.

Just like a robber, these lumps take everything you have until you feel you have nothing left. And just when you think HS has taken everything, it robs you of even more.

HS robbed me of the ability to make a living.

Data entry operators are required to sit for up to eight hours per day. Prolonged sitting is one of my HS triggers. My latest, worst flare-up, flared up quickly. Just as quickly, the pain prohibited me from working.

And not just a sit-down type of job. Oh, no, not this pain. This pain also interfered with walking and standing. The affected area is currently, overall, the size of a tennis ball. It feels like about five golf balls all jammed in there together. And that's just the thigh. The outside of the labia contains two more golf balls. When I walk and stand, they all work together to make it as painful as possible.

There are days I stay in bed, my leg propped up on a milk crate and dread those moments when I absolutely *must* go to the bathroom.

HS robbed me of social interaction.

I belonged to a writer's group. I used to get together with a friend of mine for lunch. I used to love to walk around the lake where I lived and I would have conversations with interesting people. I rode MARTA to the library to pick up books. I looked forward to the coming of spring when I could increase my exercise regimen to include walking again.

I had to stop going to the writer's group. I turned down invitations for lunch. No more visiting the library. And no walking around the lake.

I stayed inside so no one would see the pained expression on my face, or the telltale drainage on my clothing.

It got lonely.

HS robbed me of my self-esteem.

Mind you, my self-esteem never has been very high. I'm not the picture-perfect model; never have been. But I at least had enough confidence in myself to look people in the eye and know I was just as good as anyone else.

With HS, I am aware of the looks I receive when I "hobble" around in public. I'm constantly afraid the drainage will show on my clothing; I always wear black pants now. I'm also afraid of soiling furniture when I lay upon a sofa at a friend's house.

And I am acutely aware of the facial expressions people have when I explain to them what HS is. I imagine the look is akin to looks once given to lepers.

Suddenly, I don't feel as good as anyone else.

HS robbed me of my strength and energy.

Constant pain aside, HS drained me of the desire to even cook a meal. I subsisted on cheese and crackers, salads, sandwiches – anything that was quick and easy to fix and even quicker and easier to clean up after.

Ironically, a side benefit was the loss of twenty pounds. And that was without even trying. But I wouldn't recommend a dose of HS to lose weight. I would much rather have worked at weight loss with exercise. At least that would have felt better and been healthier, too.

HS robbed me of my health.

And not just my health, but also the opportunity to get *quality* health care with which to combat this illness. Without health insurance or a load of money, I cannot see those doctors who are knowledgeable about HS and treat their patients with compassion and dignity. Doctors who know I would be better equipped to deal with other situations once my distress and pain are alleviated.

Instead, I get to deal with doctors at "clinics" who hold my health hostage by demanding I conform to the patient they want me to be. Using the very words, "We won't do surgery until . . ." I jump through whatever hoops they have in place. Not to mention that not once was my depression addressed or treated.

This was not the case when I had health insurance for two previous surgeries. Heck, those two surgeons could hardly wait to get in there and take those lumps away.

What I would give to win the lottery. (Have to buy a ticket first, though, gosh darn it).

HS robbed me of my independence.

I don't drive long distances now – don't drive at all if I don't have to – because I have to prop my derriere off the seat, otherwise it is too painful to drive. I don't feel comfortable or safe driving this way, but when the cat needs food or I need toilet paper, I have little choice.

If I need something, such as Goody's headache powders to provide some relief for the pain, I often ask a friend to get some for me. In addition to the pain in my derriere, this also hurts my pride. I'm usually the one people ask for help; I'm not the one who should need it.

But the absolute worst, most vile, thing HS has robbed me of is the one thing that was the most difficult for me to earn:

HS robbed me of my freedom.

The freedom to be who I want to be, to come and go as I please, to do what I like to do.

I'll spare you the boring details and explain it this way: I spent the majority of my life trying desperately to live up to the expectations others placed upon me. I was trained to do this from the age of three.

I never succeeded.

For the last twelve, blissful years, I didn't have to do that. I was free and I would never have to live up to others' expectations again. I no longer had to explain myself or check with someone when I wanted to go somewhere. I didn't have to cave in to guilt or pressures thrust upon me by anyone else. I could make my own decisions without running them by someone else or fearing disapproval.

I swore I would never go back.

HS heard me. And said, "Think again."

Because after robbing me of my ability to support myself, my ability to interact socially and my independence, there was one last thing HS wanted: my freedom.

I fought tooth and nail. I clung to the tiniest shred of hope. I prayed, hoped and begged for a miracle. I foolishly believed a miracle was forthcoming.

But some things HS will NOT rob me of are my dignity, my will to live and my desire to beat this, this *stuff*.

As far as I am concerned, HS is an unforgivable illness.

It may rob me, but it won't defeat me. There will come a time when I will be able to rise up and reclaim all that is rightfully mine, all that I have been robbed of. And I can spit in the face of HS.

That is the day for which I live.

Three Little Words

"Have a seat."

Three little words probably stated a million times a day. Connotations may vary, but, for the most part, a cordial invitation extended in a variety of situations.

Those three little words bring terror to my heart, so much so that they almost bring me to tears.

I haven't sat in a chair for going on nine months now. And I have no idea how much longer it will be before I am able to sit in a chair again.

I have the equivalent of about five golf balls in my groin area. Not actual golf balls: I'm no masochist. But the lumps formed by Hidradenitis Suppurativa on my right thigh and the outer part of my labia are, altogether, about the size of five golf balls at this point. The pain they inflict is excruciating. They're sensitive to any pressure, as well as certain types of clothing. I'll never wear blue jeans again. Denim definitely irritates the HS. I fear sweatpants may also be out of the question.

I have no idea what I'll wear the next time I have a job interview. I'm not comfortable in dresses. Maybe a bathrobe?

Extending an invitation to sit is as natural as breathing. It indicates the person asking is comfortable with your presence and wishes to engage in conversation with you.

The person asking is not aware of how you see that chair. Through your eyes it appears to have sharp little spikes, covered with barbed wire with some broken glass thrown in for good measure.

Granted, the chair itself is not at fault. It serves its purpose well, making itself available for the parking of the derriere in a comfortable sitting position, thereby allowing a person to "take a load off."

It's the fault of those golf balls, just beneath the surface of the skin. Hard and rough, unyielding, they torment with stabbing or throbbing pain – sometimes both at the same time – itching that would drive a sane person mad and constant drainage that ruins clothing.

Healthy people take sitting with comfort and ease for granted. And with good reason. Sitting has been second nature to mankind for, oh, quite some time now. Those who do not suffer HS cannot even begin to imagine what it's like to fear a chair.

Because it does become a fear, almost a phobia to the point that I even dread hospital visits for fear of being told to "have a seat."

I used to attempt to explain why I couldn't sit in a chair. Reactions ranged from sympathetic to appalled. I admit I probably provided more details than were necessary. I try and keep the explanation simple now and merely state something to the effect that I have a condition which prohibits me from sitting.

I attempted to avoid situations where I will be asked, or required, to sit. But that is next to impossible.

Then I realized that by avoiding situations and giving footnote explanations, I was allowing an opportunity to promote awareness to pass right by. And I couldn't allow that to happen.

So, yes, when someone asks me about my health, I tell them all about HS. I compare the lumps to golf balls: That's certainly what they feel like to me. I constantly research and read articles about HS to keep up with new developments. I share that knowledge as well. I am only too happy to answer any questions about HS people pose.

As long as they don't ask me to "have a seat."

Itching For A Cure

Years ago, I used a dandruff shampoo. I had used it before and just purchased a new bottle because of an outbreak of dandruff. It's a popular brand (still on the market) and it had always worked in the past.

Once I finished washing my hair, I went to the store to pick up a few things. While standing in line to check out, I was overcome by this itching sensation from my head to my toes. It was aggravating, bordering on torturous. It felt like thousands – no, *millions* – of tiny little ants crawling all over my body.

On the drive home, the itching became so horrific I burst into tears. I couldn't get into the shower fast enough when I rushed through the door. I scrubbed for a good twenty minutes before the itching subsided.

Since the dandruff shampoo was the only thing I had used or done differently that day, I concluded (rightfully so) it was the cause of my dilemma. I never used that dandruff shampoo again. And never experienced that horrible itching again, either.

Until now, that is. Not from using any product, though I would much prefer that be the cause. At least something like that can be washed away.

HS brings an entire new level to itching. I'm grateful it doesn't itch constantly. I can handle the constant pain much better than the itching. At least I can take something for the pain. But doctors don't recommend anything for the itching. At least, not the ones I've seen.

But when it does take a notion to itch – as my mother is wont to say – it "terrifies me to death." It feels like the itching is deep within a place I simply cannot reach.

There are times, I swear, when the itching makes me wish I had long fingernails and the stamina to dig those nails into my flesh and yank out those lumps, bloody roots and all. Anything to stop the itching.

I'm not certain the cause of this itching has been addressed. I have read the itching occurs when new areas are affected or when drainage is reaching an end. However, this has not been my experience. My itching seems to occur on a whim.

It seems the symptoms of Hidradenitis Suppurativa are as unique as the individuals who suffer from them. Some people have food triggers which prompt flare-ups or itching. For me, it's stress and prolonged sitting which brings on the flare-ups. I have no idea what brings on the nightmarish itching.

A cure for this illness is long overdue. Discovered in the 1800s? Yeah, somebody's been asleep at the medical wheel, in a manner of speaking.

Modern-day doctors should, at the very least, be able to suggest something with which to combat the driving-me-absolutely-mad itching.

You would think somehow, someway, researchers could connect the dots and isolate the cause. But then, research is expensive. Heaven forbid someone should do the research just for the contribution it would make to the medical profession. Or for the relief said cure would provide hundreds of thousands of people, scratching away at they know not what.

Besides, why find a cause and a cure when there is so much more money to be made with continuous treatment and surgery? Think of the number of doctors who would miss the payments on their Jaguars. Or Porsches.

If a few doctors were subjected to a case (that's right, a CASE) of itching powder, would they then be more concerned about the effects of HS on their patients? I wonder how long it would take for someone to find a cure under those conditions.

I speak from my own personal experience. Thus far, the doctors I have dealt with have shown little compassion for my situation.

I don't wish any of the symptoms of HS on anyone. Not even those people I absolutely detest.

But I'd sure like to give them something to scratch at.

Wearing Me Out

Remember the television show *The Golden Girls*?

I specifically recall the episode where Dorothy complained of always feeling tired. Doctors shunned her complaints, told her it was merely a sign of aging. There was nothing wrong with her, as far as the doctors were concerned.

One doctor finally diagnosed Dorothy with Chronic Fatigue Syndrome, a real malady.

I know how Dorothy felt.

Even on my best days, any activity I engage in results in exhaustion.

I recently was forced to move; to vacate my bright sanctuary, trading it for an existence in a dark dungeon. I alone had to pack those belongings I couldn't part with.

Time was of the essence and I forcefully pushed myself. Combine the physical activity with the emotional stress of not wanting to move and being able to take only what was absolutely necessary and I bordered on collapse. Not just at the end of each day, but several times throughout the day.

But I had to do what I had to do in a very short amount of time.

HS attacks the autoimmune system. Not only does it weaken the body against infection, it also drains the body of the physical energy necessary to perform simple tasks. Not to mention many times it drains the body of the simple desire to even move.

Just like Dorothy in the *The Golden Girls*, doctors shun the symptom of fatigue caused by HS. Just as they do many of the other symptoms.

But the truly sad part about the fatigue is the attitude others display toward this symptom. They think I'm faking it. They think I'm just being lazy.

They think just because I have one good day in which I can actually go for a twenty minute walk that all those other days when I can hardly get out of bed are just a ploy for sympathy.

They don't understand – or maybe they don't want to understand – that the good days are anomalies. They don't get that I am just as frustrated with my illness as they are with me.

And none of this helps with the stress of the situation.

But there's not a damn thing I can do about it.

Except what I have to do. Push through the fatigue, the pain, the itching to do what must be done.

21

Pen

I'm tired just thinking about it.

For Want of a Good Night's Sleep

When you have Hidradenitis Suppurativa, sleep becomes a nodding acquaintance.

I've never really slept well to begin with. Sleep apnea and bathroom usage are companions that awaken me a number of times during the night.

They have a new companion to help with the job: HS.

Except HS is a far superior sleep inhibitor than the other two combined. In addition to awakening me from a semi-peaceful slumber, it prevents me from sleeping at all.

Normally, I sleep on my left side. Thanks to a deviated septum (yeah, I'm pretty much a mess) it's the most comfortable position in which to sleep.

Now, there is no position of comfort. Lumps on my right thigh and the outer portion of my labia rub against each other providing constant discomfort and outright pain. Sleeping on either side is next to impossible.

In the early stages of this latest flare-up, I could lie face down across my bed and sleep pretty well that way. Over time, however, the HS spread. To the front. Lying face down is no longer an option.

As a last resort, I have taken to propping my right leg on top of a milk crate with a pillow or blanket on top to prevent chafing from the plastic crate. It sometimes alleviates the pressure, discomfort and pain long enough for me to sleep in short bursts.

It doesn't always work. There are times when I attempt to grab a couple zzzs only to be thwarted by the incessant pain in that area. No position on earth provides relief. And if it isn't the pain keeping me awake, it's that blasted itching.

I cannot recall the last time I slept a full eight hours. I am relegated to napping when the pain and itching are at a minimum. Some days I function on less than two hours of sleep at a time, a few times during the course of a 24-hour period.

Some days – though rarely and with the help of some Goody's headache powders – I sleep blissfully for several hours at a stretch. Ironically, that sleep occurs during the day and I am subsequently up all night long.

Not that being up all night long is a bad thing. I get some writing done and I'm able to catch an episode of *Quantum Leap*. Sadly, these are the highlights of my life these days.

The human body requires sleep. It's a way to reboot the system, revive and refresh physical energy and mental capacity.

When the sleep pattern gets out of whack, so does everything else.

As with the itching sensation, this, too, has not been addressed by the medical profession. Of course, the first thing doctors do is prescribe sleep medication.

Sure, that's the ticket. It's so much easier to prescribe another pill than it is to find a cure or actually treat the problem. While sleep medication may work, it's still a quick fix and not a treatment.

It's as though HS mimics several different maladies. It has the chronic pain of dislocated spinal discs, throws in the constant itching of allergic reactions or rashes, adds the disfiguring effects of shingles and, for good measure, it brings isolation and depression to the party.

By the same token, the medical profession mimic treatment. Pain medication, sleep medication, depression medication – all with side effects, mind you – treating the symptoms instead of finding the cause and subsequent cure. To add to the consternation, the itching is completely ignored.

Please forgive my blasting the medical profession. I haven't come across many medical personnel lately who are professional.

Chronic pain, itching to the point of insanity, constant drainage that ruins my clothing, lack of sleep . . . and people wonder why I'm cranky.

No Sex Life

At the age of 54, I have a confession to make: I have never had an intimate relationship.

Not from a lack of desire and certainly not from a lack of trying.

There were a number of issues involved in my shying away from intimacy. Being overweight, body image was an issue. Being an introvert didn't help. Expectations were another matter: my own expectations as well as those placed upon me.

But the biggest issue that kept from allowing me to engage in sexual activity was Hidradenitis Suppurativa.

It was bad enough I had to endure it. I wasn't about to allow anyone else to get near it. Not to mention the pain of HS made even the thought of sexual activity painful.

I always hoped for an intimate relationship. Finding someone who wouldn't be disgusted with my body and its afflictions was one of my most ardent and secret desires.

After my second surgery, I abandoned that hope.

I realize a relationship is possible: intimacy is not limited to physical contact. It is possible to have a fulfilling relationship without sex.

I would be all for that. Except, at this point, I'm just not certain I'm up for it.

I realize it is my own self-consciousness which holds me back from having an intimate relationship. It has played a large role in that respect.

But the psychological damage is done. I cannot bear the thought of another person – except a doctor or nurse – viewing the afflicted area.

My self-esteem and self-worth have been submarined by this disease. It's a lot of baggage to carry and a huge burden for anyone to take on in a relationship. There is a certain degree of unfairness to both parties.

And I can't blame anyone else for not wanting to take on the baggage or the burden. I'd heave it off the side of a bridge if I could. Abandon it on the railroad tracks.

It would take years of therapy for me to unravel and deal with all that baggage. I certainly don't expect anyone to wait around while I do.

They say you don't miss what you've never had. I wish that were true. Just because I've never had that kind of love, doesn't mean I haven't imagined it.

But I rarely imagine it these days. The pain interferes with even the desire to imagine an intimate relationship.

It is yet another side effect of HS: keeping intimacy at bay. Sometimes, even keeping friends at arm's length fares better for the HS sufferer.

I suppose on the upside, finding someone with whom to spend my life is one less thing to worry about.

I'll not be thanking HS for that anytime soon.

No Jury Will Convict

If a person were inflicting this much pain upon my body, I would use whatever I had at my disposal to try and stop them. Pencil, pen, fork, knife, baseball bat, cement block: Whatever I grabbed I would swing for all I was worth until the assailant was a bloody pulp.

I would be acting on the assumption that the assailant is assaulting me with the intent to kill. Instinct takes over; my mind and body respond with fight or flight instincts. Self-preservation kicks in and I do what I must to save my own life. Nature supplies us with these instincts in order to preserve the human race overall.

No jury in the world would convict me.

It's a little more difficult to fight an invisible assailant, especially when that invisible assailant attacks you from within your own body.

You can't very well take a club or a butcher knife to Hidradenitis Suppurativa, though tempting it may be. Self-inflicted wounds are frowned upon, even when they are inflicted against an enemy.

HS delivers pain that never stops. Alleviation of pain through medication,

30

soaking, warm compresses or finally being able to find a comfortable position are only temporary. The pain doesn't go away. It's still there, beneath the surface throbbing away.

Throb. Throb. Throb. PUNCH! Throb. Throb. PUNCH!

Your assailant just blindsided you with a baseball bat. You have nothing with which to fight off this assailant. The best you can do is clench your fists and grit your teeth to keep from crying out or screaming. If you cry out or scream, people look at you as if you should be in a rubber room.

How do you combat an enemy too cowardly to show its face?

You do what you must. You sleep. A lot. You go to doctor's appointments and do what you're told, even if you don't want to. You hit things that don't hit back: your car hood, a pillow, your closet door. You cry until your tear ducts are as dry as the Sahara. You vent to your best friend. You find a comfortable position in which to recline and you don't move for hours, no matter how hungry or thirsty you get. Because if you eat or drink, that means you'll have to get up sometime to go to the bathroom. Going to the bathroom only exacerbates the pain.

You lose weight.

You hope, you wish and you pray each and every day, a hundred times over, for a miracle, any miracle that will take away this pain. You accept and endure the disappointment that follows when no miracle is offered.

You lose hope.

And the fight rages on inside you.

But you keep fighting this invisible assailant because you are determined to defeat such a cowardly enemy. You will not give in to its ravages, no matter what it uses to beat you down, you will defeat it. And you will use everything at your disposal to beat it down and overcome it.

No jury in the world will convict you.

The Emotional Impact of
Hidradenitis Suppurativa

Hidradenitis Suppurativa attacks the human body physically.

If only it stopped there.

Some illnesses which plague the human body cannot be seen, even on the skin. Most cancers occur within the body.

HS itself cannot be displayed due to the locations in which it occurs: beneath armpits and breasts, along the groin and buttocks. It makes it invisible to everyone except the one suffering from it. And, of course, doctors and nurses.

But HS is a greedy illness with a voracious appetite. It wants not only to disfigure the human body physically, it also wants to destroy the emotional and mental aspects of its victim.

Depression is an all-too-common side effect. Dealing with chronic pain 24 hours a day, 7 days a week will do that. As do the feelings of hopelessness and isolation. For some, even family and friends refuse to acknowledge what we are going through, based simply upon the fact that the physical ravages are not evident to their eyes.

Loss of energy, strength accompany the chronic pain. Ea drains the body of precious immune system is weakened as mental health. One is left feeling destitute.

Self-worth flees at the ad Going from being a productive society to an indigent individu person's sense of self-worth.

If that doesn't accomplish the also the fact that people are not or how debilitating it is. There i compassion by those in t profession, many of whom don' HS is or how to treat it. And th who choose to not treat it.

The lack of compassion f friends and others is comparable the overall lack of compassion ir community.

A person begins to see the failure, incapable of taking care o unable to dig their way out of th and the deep pit in which they find

At times the temptation to giv Throw in the towel, check out pe

There is no judgment on those this option. Dealing with the chr an illness without a cure is daur not reflect upon anyone's strength of character when they choose to no longer deal with such a horrific illness.

Those who continue dealing with it are no stronger or no weaker than those who do not. Some of us simply do not know what else to do but awaken each day with some slender hope that things will eventually get better.

While this may sound easy, it is not. Because each day is the same: We are still in pain, we are still depressed, we are still isolated.

Yet we still hope.

The true challenge lies in not allowing HS to completely destroy that hope.

Stress, the Ultimate Trigger

Stress is a dangerous thing. It can lead to heart attacks, strokes, illness . . . and it is one of the biggest triggers of my Hidradenitis Suppurativa.

I have read a few articles and writing by others that cite stress as a contributor to HS.

While I can certainly vouch for that, stress is one of the major triggers of my own HS.

I am fortunate that I do not suffer high blood pressure. On the contrary, my blood pressure tends to run a little on the low side. Since no doctor has ever addressed that, I assume it's a good thing.

I learned a long time ago not to stress over the little stuff. Laid off from a job? No sweat. Job search and write until I have another one. Car broke down? Piece o'cake. I lived on the MARTA rail line. I could hop the bus to a train station.

All of that changed with this latest flare-up.

Finances are a huge stress factor for me. Currently being completely without finances or the means to generate income is about to send me over the edge.

Couple that with a family lacking in understanding and compassion . . . let's just say I'm about ready for a padded cell.

Not to mention I'm almost ready to take a butcher knife to these godforsaken lumps.

It's all about those expectations I mentioned before. I did the taking-care-of-Mom thing for fifteen years after my father passed away. Mind you, my mother is no invalid. But she has never driven a car in her life. Someone must take her grocery shopping, to Walmart, to her doctor's appointments.

I was the one expected to do this. Even though her house was filled with other adults capable of doing the same thing, her two sons and their live-in girlfriends never once offered. When asked, there was always an excuse.

There are still excuses. And I am still expected to do these things. I knew it would be this way when I had to move into my mother's house.

It doesn't matter how many times I tell these people how painful it is for me to drive my car. I have to raise my derriere so it doesn't touch the seat. It is not a comfortable way to drive, nor does it feel safe. There's only so long I can do that before my legs begin to shake. But none of that matters. The important thing is that Mom gets what she wants.

To refuse to do what is expected of me only exacerbates the stress. Refusal results in tantrums: the tossing of dishware onto the table, the slamming of cabinet doors, a cold shoulder. To inquire about what is wrong makes matters worse: a cold shoulder for days on end.

We are not a family who talks things out. Nor are we close. Never have been. Never will be.

I realize this may sound as though I am whining and maybe I am.

But I'm trying to illustrate the role stress plays in the life of an HS sufferer. Being in a stressful situation inhibits the body's healing process. Stress weakens the immune system. Worse, it also weakens the resolve and determination of a person to overcome the illness. It kills the hope of being happy and healthy.

It is little wonder that, with each passing day, I feel worse. The stress of caring for two people is more than one person can handle. Especially when one person carries all the stigma of HS.

I sleep as much as possible to alleviate the stress. I write. I go to the library to use the Internet. I read.

That's about all I can do under the circumstances.

And hope neither the stress, nor the HS kills me.

In a Tunnel Dark

Why can't I find a compassionate doctor willing to help?

You're not worth it.

Why won't someone find a cure for Hidradenitis Suppurativa?

You're not worth it.

That's the HS talking. That voice is very loud and it gives the same answer to a string of questions: *You're not worth it.*

When you're in a dark tunnel, you begin to believe what the voice says, because there is no light to contradict the darkness.

Depression is almost a constant companion for those who suffer HS. It begins upon learning there is no cure for this illness. It will plague you throughout your life, so count on periodic surgeries and hospital stays.

Isolation then creeps in. Embarrassment and shame about things over which you have no control: drainage which soils clothing, walking funny or being unable to use your arms due to the pain, not being able to sit for the same reason. There is shame over the illness itself, virtually an unknown entity to the public and the medical profession alike.

Compounding the isolation are those lacking in compassion: employers, coworkers, friends and family. Employers have little tolerance for employees missing time from work due to illness. All too often, HS results in job loss. Coworkers don't understand why you're not functioning up to par, even after you explain things to them.

Friends don't understand – and some take outright offense – when you decline invitations to lunch, dinner, the movies or similar outings due to chronic pain, excessive drainage or both. Slowly, some of those friends just . . . drift away.

Family, however, is the worst. Not all families are compassionate, understanding or supportive. There are family members who believe you're "faking it" for attention or sympathy. Other members blame you for this condition in one way or another, as if it is your fault because of weight or lifestyle or some other such ridiculous reason.

It always hurts worst when it comes from your family.

Combine isolation with chronic pain and drainage, little support from loved ones and those in the medical field, toss in little hope of ever being completely rid of this condition and you get one gigantic case of depression. This is elephant-sized depression sitting on your shoulders; so heavy and burdensome that you buckle beneath the weight.

Holding on for one more day is often an Olympian feat. It is difficult to throw off the depression, equally difficult to dig your way out of it.

This depression infiltrates your every waking moment. Self-worth gets flushed down the toilet. Of course it does: You are not a productive member of society, your friends have fled, and your family thinks you're just bucking for disability. Basically, you're a piece of crap.

That's when the HS really starts to rock'n'roll. It has you just where it wants you.

But you fight. You fight by sleeping through the worst of the depression. You fight by making quilts. You fight by writing, daydreaming, watching television or DVDs, reading books, listening to music or having a cryfest in your pillow. Whatever it takes to get you through this depression because you'll be damned if HS is going to win.

Sometimes, the HS does win. I do not blame or judge those who choose to leave this world because of HS. It is as daunting as it is debilitating. To say I haven't considered doing the same would be an outright lie.

I feel for them. And I mourn for them, even though I do not know them.

To be dragged down into that dark tunnel and to remain there not knowing when you may see the light of day is something I hope most people never have to experience.

To those who do experience that tunnel allow me to say this: You are worth it. There will be a light. Do what you must until it arrives.

Because, one day, there will be hands – helping hands, healing hands – reaching into that tunnel to bring you to that light or bring that light to you.

Hope. There must always be hope. Find it wherever you can. Cling to it with all your strength.

You are worth it.

Self-Imposed Isolation

When prisoners act out, they are placed in isolation.

When patients carry contagious illnesses, they are placed in isolation.

When a person suffers from Hidradenitis Suppurativa, isolation becomes a way of life.

The effects of shame and embarrassment play vital roles in the lives of people who suffer from HS.

HS sufferers have no reason to be embarrassed or ashamed. The human body is susceptible to all manner of ailments, none of which a person wishes to endure: cancer, Parkinson's, Gehrig's . . . and Hidradenitis Suppurativa.

The perception society has of the human body is based upon what people see in advertising, on television and in movies. Healthy, super thin, clear-skinned beautiful women and ruggedly handsome men define what the rest of us should look like. We are inundated with those images to the point our expectations of the human body are buried within our subconscious, even those of us who try and not think that way.

So if a human body falls short of those expectations or falls victim to a chronic, debilitating and disfiguring illness such as HS, there is cause for shame and embarrassment according to society's perception.

The stigma of experiencing an illness unknown to most people follows the HS sufferer no matter where she or he goes. Explaining HS and its effects to people garners little sympathy. Most look at you as though you're someone best avoided, as though you are contagious, when nothing could be further from the truth.

Excessive drainage and constant pain escalate the senses of shame and embarrassment. The drainage is often malodorous and soils clothing. Few of us wear shorts in the summertime for fear of drainage escaping whatever we have in place to catch it. But the drainage also seeps onto clothing beneath the arms and breasts, rendering some clothing unsalvageable regardless of numerous launderings.

Constant pain limits movement. For some, it interferes with the use of their arms. Lifting something as small as a loaf of bread causes pain and irritation. For others, standing, walking and sitting cause a great deal of pain.

So the HS sufferer declines invitations to meet with friends, to go out to lunch or dinner or to go see a movie.

It doesn't take long for friends to stop calling or offering moral support.

Our self-esteem and feeling of self-worth declines along with our health.

Those of us who suffer from HS hide from the rest of the world. Because the rest of the world sends us subtle messages that we are not to be seen. We are not to be acknowledged.

And we receive those messages. And we believe them. Because those messages come from people who matter to us. And they come from ourselves as well.

And, yes, most of us impose isolation upon ourselves. Because it is painful to see the looks of disgust we get should the drainage show. It is painful to know our friends are ashamed of us: We are ashamed ourselves.

It takes a strong individual to endure the isolation.

It takes an even stronger person to ignore society's perception and to continue a daily routine, not allowing what others think to persuade our own self-image.

But the human ego is often more fragile than the human body. Many people are acutely aware of how others see them; incredibly perceptive to looks and feelings of disapproval and disgust.

Truth be told, everyone wants approval, whether from employers, family or friends. Their disapproval pierces like a knife.

So when an HS sufferer experiences those looks and attitudes of disapproval and disgust, it drives down their self-esteem and self-worth.

It is a never-ending battle.

The physical battle is difficult enough in and of itself. The battle to maintain a positive, healthy outlook is compounded by the shame and embarrassment encountered upon stepping outside one's door.

So, self-imposed isolation. It simply makes dealing with the HS easier. No explanations. No dirty looks, no disapproval, no looks of disgust. No rejection from those who mean the most to us.

It makes dealing with HS easier. But it also makes it more difficult. Dealing with any illness alone is an overwhelming task. Dealing with an illness with no known cause, no cure and about which few people are educated is a Herculean task. It is a task no one would willingly take on.

Few people understand this. HS sufferers didn't ask for this illness.

But rather than face those people, it's just better to be alone.

Weight Loss the HS Way

I have struggled with my weight all my life. I was born overweight and pretty much stayed that way.

As with most overweight people, I've had my ups and downs. I'd lose about twenty pounds and then put thirty right back on.

I did manage to lose down to 170 and maintained that weight for some time.

Then I had my heart attack. I lost ten pounds while in the hospital for five days.

I kept that off, too.

Then Hidradenitis Suppurativa came to town.

Being unable to work, well that means you're not able to purchase food, either. If you don't eat, you definitely lose weight.

But even during the times when friends brought me some food or when a neighbor generously purchased food for me with her food stamps, I didn't eat much.

It wasn't so much that I wasn't hungry or didn't have an appetite. The physical act of cooking a meal was exhausting. I never realized how tiring it was to scramble up a couple of eggs. Or to bake some chicken in the oven while boiling broccoli on the stove.

This is not an exaggeration. The pain, the inflammation, the drainage while doing something as simple as washing dishes took enough out of me to warrant a four-hour nap to recuperate.

So I drastically changed my eating habits. I went for the most simple of foods: sandwiches, toast, salads, crackers. Quick and easy to fix, quick and easy to clean up after. I used paper towels instead of plates so I had fewer dishes to wash. I kept crackers nearby so I could eat a few when I felt hungry. I didn't eat much. Exercising to burn off calories was out of the question.

I suspect HS itself burned off a few calories, just from the energy of its aggressive invasion of my body.

It didn't take long for the adjustment in eating habits to reflect on the scale. I was surprised one day in March to see I had lost twenty pounds since December.

Health issues put me down to 140 pounds.

Though I could still stand to lose about another 15 pounds, this is the least I have weighed in my adulthood.

This is not how I wanted to lose weight. It is not a healthy way to lose weight. I much prefer to eat sensibly and walk it off.

I admit I've not been very good at doing that in the past. But I have a new perspective on weight loss and exercise. You never appreciate something as much as when it is taken away from you.

When I finally get rid of this round of HS, I will no longer take for granted the ability to walk without pain. Or ride an exercise bike or work out in any other way without the interference of pain and inflammation.

People congratulate me for losing twenty pounds. They don't understand the weight loss is due to illness and not a healthy lifestyle. Skin hangs loose from my arms and thighs. I do what I can by lifting five pound weights in each hand as often as possible, but I fear it is not enough to tone those arms.

There is little I can do about the legs since that is where the lumps are. I sometimes attempt to walk. I love to walk. I used to walk a lot around the lake where I used to live. Now I get to walk beside a train track.

But if I walk one day, I end up paying for it for the next two days with swelling and increased pain.

I do what I can, when I can.

Weight loss due to health issues is not something to be happy about.

I always wanted to lose weight. But I never wanted to get sick to do it.

So, please, don't congratulate me.

Moral Support Works Wonders

I don't expect people to understand what I'm going through. Unless they experience it themselves, they can't truly understand.

But is it too much to ask for a little moral support?

I have one friend – my best friend, bless her heart – who calls me each and every night to see how I am. Or just to talk.

Then there are those people in my life who insist I get a job. Even a part-time job.

I'd love to be able to work a part-time job. At least it would bring in some type of income. But I seriously doubt I would be able to stick with a job – any job – for more than a week at the most. Sometimes I barely make it through an ordinary day without feeling like collapsing.

I've tried my best to convince my friends to help promote my books. ANY sales would boost my morale, if nothing else.

They share what I post about my books. Without an Internet connection, I can't post anything. So it doesn't get shared. But my friends don't take it upon themselves to post anything.

I realize everyone has their own lives. I'm not faulting them for that. But their lack of promoting my books on their own makes me feel as if they don't even give me a thought.

Another friend gave me two fundraisers in an attempt to bring in some type of finances. Neither of them brought in enough funds to help, nor did either of them get attention or additional support.

Ironically, I was expected to do all the promotion for both fundraisers. At the time, I had to lie face down on the floor to access my computer. When the HS reached a certain level, it became painful to do even that. So I didn't do it very often.

My friend couldn't seem to understand why I wasn't promoting the fundraisers 24/7.

And now, the family situation. I am expected to care for our 88-year-old mother. My health is not on anyone's priority list. Not even my own at this point.

Moral support. What does that even look like?

Hugs are a great place to start. A shoulder to cry on would be tremendous.

And while words are wonderful things, actions are more powerful.

Picking up the phone to call and just chat. Asking if there is anything I need, instead of telling me to call you if I need something. If you know me at all, you know I hate to ask.

How about checking some books out at the library for me? You know I've been dying to read the latest James Rollins novel. It's difficult for me to get to and from the library.

Tell me it's okay that I can't work and be a productive member of society rather than continuously putting pressure on me to get a job. Sure, it'd be nice to make money, but when I think of how much more pain I would have to endure to perform the job, I cringe.

Oh, and if you're going to do a fundraiser FOR me, you really need to take on the majority of the responsibility of organizing and getting the word out. Shouldn't you? I mean, isn't that how a fundraiser is supposed to work?

And don't get pissy when I don't put the milk container back exactly as you had it. Or if I'm too tired or in too much pain to take you to the grocery store.

But, most of all, promote my books. Tell everyone you know how much you enjoy reading my work. Encourage them to purchase a copy. And tell them to tell all their friends.

My morale is vastly improved with even one book sale. Enough book sales (it truly wouldn't take many) would get me to a real doctor so I can get the surgery I need to resume a healthy and somewhat normal life. Even if it is only for another four years before the next flare-up occurs.

Is any of this too much to ask? Or do I not have the right to make the request?

Maybe I am not being clear about my requests.

Asking for moral support really shouldn't even be a question. Especially from those who care about you.

Yet it seems to be the most difficult thing people can do.

Treat HS Patients with a little more Compassion, Why Doncha?

The medical profession is supposed to be one of compassion.

Unless you suffer from Hidradenitis Suppurativa (HS).

Allow me to state, I haven't had the best experiences dealing with medical professionals when it comes to HS.

My latest flare-up in October of last year sent me to the emergency room by December. I survived a heart attack in 2013 and in December of last year, I began experiencing pressure in my chest and just a little twinge of pain. Since I was still breathing and walking around, I asked a friend to take me to the emergency room.

There, my heart was checked out immediately. All was well. That was a relief.

Now to see a doctor about my HS.

When you go to an emergency room when the emergency is not life-threatening, there is no place to lie down. At least, there wasn't any place in this emergency room.

So I was forced – literally *forced* – to sit for seven hours as people who came in long after me were ushered in to see a doctor. I told the nurses on duty I was in excruciating pain due to the location of the lumps and could not sit. But was anyone compassionate about that? Of course not. I kept asking how much longer it would be, would it be soon, is there anything you can do? I was told to sit and wait.

Another emergency room visit in March to a different hospital. Again, not life-threatening. I informed the nurses I couldn't sit. I was told it would be a seven-hour wait.

I was elated to find a short bench and proceeded to lie upon it.

Every five minutes I was harassed by a nurse: "Sit up!" "You can't lie down!" "Other patients need to sit here."

"But I told you it is painful for me to sit!"
"Sit up!"

I felt like weeping. I felt like throwing a tantrum. But I knew that would either get me kicked out, land me in the psych ward or get me signed up for Anger Management classes.

So for quite some time, I stood, walked around, waited for the bench to become available again and slipped right back down on it.

The harassment continued without end.

Where was the compassion? Especially from nurses who, usually, are more compassionate than doctors?

This is an emergency room. Yes, I realize my emergency is not life-threatening, according to your definitions. But my body is in distress, whether you can see it or not. If a patient tells you, "I cannot sit," what? Do you think he or she is kidding? Being lazy? Do you think I'm some vagrant who came in off the street just to lie down? I have a damn good reason for not sitting.

I would *love* to be able to sit in one of these chairs, lady, but that would be subjecting *myself* to an enormous amount of pain. Why would I want to do that? What about that don't you understand?

Is it a matter of ignorance? Are emergency room personnel uneducated about the symptoms and unique problems associated with HS? Or do they choose to harass patients because of some idiotic hospital protocols? Why would a hospital have such protocols in place as to force a patient to *painfully* endure seven or eight hours of waiting?

A hospital is supposed to *alleviate* pain, not inflict it. Nurses are supposed to *soothe*, not be Nazis about whether or not you're sitting, lying down or hanging from the rafters. (Okay, the latter I couldn't do anyway, but I would do it if it alleviated the pain).

The lack of compassion and under-standing of medical personnel towards people with HS is shameful, neglectful and inexcusable. There is no reason to harass someone because of the pain he or she is in. There is no reason to harass someone simply because you feel you have the right to do so or because there's some stupid hospital policy that gives you the authority to do so.

Just because you *have* the right, doesn't *make* it right.

And that is what treatment of HS is really all about: whether or not those in the medical profession choose to do the RIGHT thing and treat HS patients with compassion.

Protocols be damned.

Death Would be a Relief

I get it. I completely understand.

All hope is lost. The pain is chronic as are other symptoms. There is no relief in sight.

And a person decides she or he has had enough. A person determines that one more day in this plight is intolerable.

And chooses to take their leave of this world.

Oh, yes. I get it. I grieve for those whose pain and desolation take them to that point. But I also understand it.

To say the thought of committing suicide has not crossed my mind would be an outright lie. Many times during these last nine months, it has occurred to me that, in death, there would be no more pain.

No self-esteem, feeling worthless, feeling like I don't matter, whether I live or die makes no difference, drainage, pain, pain and more pain. Throw in the callous attitude of the medical professionals I've dealt with, the constant reminder that I'm poor and undeserving of medical treatment, and just the damned inability to sit in a chair stirs up anguish which only exacerbates the problem.

Some days it is more difficult than others to hold on for just one more day.

So, yes, the thought of sleep – blissful, painless, forever sleep – is an idea worth giving serious consideration.

When I am at my lowest, I confess, there is little that improves my mood. My best friend, with all good intentions, attempts to lighten things, maybe make me laugh. But my desire and energy to laugh and look on the good side has fled. During those moments, there is no good side.

I've told people "trade places with me" when they look at me with doubt. While they sit in a chair without pain or walk instead of hobble, I'm gritting my teeth to keep from screaming from the pain shooting through my thigh and I tell them, "trade places with me."

There are many people I encounter who would not have lasted as long as I have. They would have thrown in the towel months ago.

Giving up is so much easier. Just let go and slip away while the pain becomes a thing of the past. No more worries, no more being a burden, no more responsibilities. No more begging to be admitted to the hospital, no more callous doctors. All gone. Facing whatever comes after, for better or worse.

Yet, I don't give up.

This is not a testimony to my strength or my stubbornness. I simply don't know what else to do except continue waking each morning with some slender hope that something will change today. Something will get better. Maybe today there will be a miracle.

I have prayed, hoped, begged and pleaded each and every day for nine months for that miracle.

But miracles don't happen these days. Particularly for someone like me: someone who has been overlooked for the whole of my life.

Some days the desire to check out is stronger than others. Those days I usually stay in bed, barely moving for fear I may act upon that desire. I spend a good deal of time inside my own head, engaging in daydreams of a healthier time.

I'm not looking for accolades for my perseverance or strength, determination or will to live. Those don't even come into play.

So what is it that keeps me going? What prevents me from taking an overdose to check out of this world?

Just one thing: I have books to write. I have stories to tell. And I refuse to go out until I have exhausted each and every one of the ideas circulating in my head.

Maybe I will not be a successful author in my own lifetime. At least I will leave behind a part of myself and, one day, others will come to appreciate what I have left behind.

They probably won't realize what I went through to leave it behind. But that doesn't really matter.

Someday. That's what really matters. Someday.

Someday is what I hold on for. It's all I have.

Like Turning on a Faucet

Drainage. Anyone who suffers Hidra-denitis Suppurativa knows all about it.

For starters, it stinks. In every meaning of the word. It smells horrible. But it also stinks for other reasons.

It soils clothing and furniture alike. To the point that clothing must be discarded and precautions must be taken to prevent ruining furniture. Even incontinent underwear and feminine hygiene pads cannot capture all the drainage. Towels or other cloth must be used to protect furniture.

Then there's the embarrassment of having the crap run down your leg or sides, depending upon the location of the abscesses. It is rare that I wear shorts in public. Likewise, I imagine a good many HS sufferers do not wear tank tops or short sleeves. After all, we must not subject others to the disgrace of the drainage.

With the help of antibiotics – Bactrim in particular – I experienced the bliss of drastically decreased drainage. It was wonderful not to change the pads every half hour.

Unfortunately, when the Bactrim ran out, the drainage returned with a vengeance. It was like turning on a faucet. It flows freely and changing of the pads and underwear is more frequent.

It gets costly. But I know of no other way to keep the nasty discharge from ruining everything it touches.

Having a doctor drain the things is of little use. The size, location and number of lumps guarantees drainage will continue until these monsters are removed. Thus far, no doctor has offered to drain the monstrosities anyway.

Getting more Bactrim is currently out of the question. This requires a clinic visit with cost which I do not have at the moment. Fortunately, the Bactrim is free at Publix. Without a prescription, I cannot get it right now.

So I deal with the drainage as best I can. Compared to the pain, the drainage is an annoyance. But it's a big annoyance.

One day this will come to an end, somehow, someway. In the meantime, I may have to start wearing a bucket between my legs.

Won't that be lovely?

Who Needs Pads?

I guess I still do.

I thought I was over it. The time during my life when my menstrual cycle stopped, I celebrated. No more unexpected visits, no more cramps, and, best of all, no more buying those feminine hygiene products. Finally, I could save some money.

Ten years later, I stand in the checkout line with two packages of pads in my cart.

It's not the monthly monster that forces me to purchase pads in bulk. It's the monster taking up permanent residence in my groin that requires the use of pads. They come in handy for preventing the drainage from Hidradenitis Suppurativa from completely soiling clothing and furniture alike. Or, at least, the pad captures most of it. Most of the time.

I'm sure the manufacturers of these products never dreamed they would be used for such a purpose. I'm also certain if they knew the true versatility of feminine hygiene products they'd probably charge more for them.

I often wonder what the cashier thinks as s/he rings up the packages. It's obvious I'm past that age. Maybe they think I'm purchasing them for a daughter. The only daughter I have is a four-legged feline who wouldn't appreciate having a feminine hygiene pad attached to her tail.

I used to feel as though I single-handedly kept the feminine hygiene companies in business.

But then I read a few stories of women suffering from Hidradenitis Suppurativa who also use the pads for the same reason I do.

I guess I'm not the only genius to come up with that idea.

It's annoying, but it's a necessity.

Even more annoying, I use the pads in conjunction with incontinence underwear.

This may seem like overkill. In truth, it still isn't enough.

Why not just use the incontinent underwear? There are a few reasons.

First, the underwear is far more expensive than the pads. Drainage is such that I would require replacing the underwear each time I used the bathroom. I simply cannot afford to keep that much incontinence underwear stocked up.

Second, due to the location of my HS, the plastic lining along the sides of the underwear tend to irritate the affliction. The pads are used to cover up the plastic and capture the drainage along the side.

Sadly, with all this precaution, the drainage still manages to run down my leg from time to time, depending upon how ambitious it is upon a particular day.

Third, I simply can no longer wear regular underwear. Drainage soiled every pair I had to the point of being unsalvageable. The elastic along the sides also irritated the HS. Regular underwear doesn't have a plastic lining outside to trap the drainage, ergo, more soiling of clothing and furniture.

Not to mention I can't afford to keep replacing regular underwear, either. Or to keep them laundered. Too many launderings and they begin to fall apart anyway.

It is not a pleasant situation. But it is often necessary to do unpleasant things for our own protection.

I just hope that if anyone ever markets these products to HS sufferers, they don't raise the prices.

HS-induced Dream

I don't dream often. When I do dream, I rarely recall the dream. Even when I can recall a dream, it makes no sense. Interpretation eludes me. Most of the time, I forget about the dream and move on.

But this dream, I cannot forget. It occurred during a very difficult period for me. My HS was doing its worst. Every move was painful. I spent hours sleeping on my sofa, only moving when it was absolutely necessary.

May 1, 2016

I am walking along a road with a group of friends, none of whom I recognize. We need to get back to my car. My car is in Athens. I tell my friends this.

In the dream, I am carrying an armload of stuff, more than I should be carrying. My friends do not lighten my burden or offer to help.

We come to a fork in the road. In order to get to my car, I must take the left fork because it is the one that goes to Athens. I start walking the left fork. It is difficult, because it is painful to walk and hard to walk with my arms full of the stuff I'm carrying.

My friends continue walking along the right fork. I hope they see me and realize their mistake. They don't. They continue walking. And they're talking and laughing, oblivious to the fact that I am not with them.

I remember thinking, "I told them the car was in Athens." I see them walking along the other fork and hope they see me.

In the dream, I visualize them seeing me and realizing their mistake. They rush over to me, apologetic, and begin unloading my burden, each sharing in it so it isn't so heavy.

But this does not happen.

I am left to walk alone, with my pain and my burden, to get to where I need to be.

This dream doesn't require much interpretation. I felt abandoned by my friends, it's that simple. My friends have helped me as much as they can. Everyone is dealing with stuff right now, most of it financial. It's just that the help they gave was not enough to help me dig my way out of the pit HS put me in.

It isn't their fault and I do not hold them accountable for my ill health. I appreciate their efforts. My friends are doing their best and I'm not saying their best isn't good enough.

But I do long for my friends to see and acknowledge the burden under which I struggle. I wish they would at least try and lighten the load, even if just a little.

It doesn't have to be with money. Taking the time to call and actually listen is as important, if not more so, than paying the bills.

The dream pretty much speaks for itself.

But I don't want any more dreams. Living through it is nightmare enough.

Commercial for HS Medication

Haven't seen it yet? That's because there isn't one as of this writing.

But I can imagine what one would look like.

I see those commercials for medications for depression and other illnesses. Some of them are downright scary.

When you're peddling a pill for depression and one of the side effects is "suicidal thoughts," I really have to wonder about that.

Sure, the pharmaceutical companies have to cover their derrieres but why would you want to market a drug that *contributes* to an illness?

Why, to make money, of course.

I would think the pharmaceutical corporations would make haste to develop a drug to treat HS: more money in their coffers. It would be best, of course, to know more about the illness before developing a drug to treat it, but that's never stopped the moneymakers before.

Visualize with me as I write the first ever television commercial for HS medication.

We see a woman curled up on her bed. A voice over says, "Do you suffer from

72

Hidradenitis Suppurativa? Does constant drainage cause you embarrassment? Ask your doctor about XYZ pills. XYZ is not a cure, but decreases drainage, pain and inflammation caused by HS. Side effects have been known to cause nausea, dizziness, drowsiness, depression, sudden and unexpected flare ups, increased drainage and inflammation, irritability, loneliness, bloating, swelling of joints, memory loss, and thoughts of suicide. You may grow extra appendages or your hair or eyes may change color while taking XYZ. Call your doctor immediately if you experience any of these symptoms while taking XYZ."

As the narrator speaks, the woman gets up from the bed and goes about her daily life: walking in the park, grocery shopping, playing Frisbee with the dog, preparing a meal. She's smiling. She's happy. None of those nasty side effects are evident.

Of course, she's an actress and has no clue what HS really is.

People suffering an illness – and HS sufferers in particular – can't seem to catch a break. A drug that treats an illness is just as likely to be as harmful as it is helpful.

I'm anxious for a cure for HS. But I'm just as wary about what someone cooks up for the cure. How many side effects can we expect? And what will those side effects be? Will they contribute to HS rather than decrease the illness?

I understand the side effects warning on medications. Developing medication to treat a specific illness is a roll of the dice. The symptoms for HS vary as much as the individuals it afflicts. What works for some may not work for others. Different drugs affect different people in different ways.

But there will come a day – though I'm sure it's still a long way off – when there will be advertisements on television and in magazines for the latest "miracle" drug to treat HS.

Just pay attention to the side effects.

Where is the Help?

When there is a catastrophe on the news, people – complete strangers – step up to help. They give clothing, money, food to help those in need.

When refugees come to the United States they are given free housing, free food and free health care. Yes, those refugees have a harder life than we do. I'm not saying they don't deserve the special treatment. Even if those benefits are temporary, it's still more than American citizens receive.

I am saying that there are American citizens who fall by the wayside in the effort to support those refugees. If you are a homeless veteran, there is little available to you. If you lose your home due to illness, no one pitches in to help.

If you suffer from a debilitating illness and you're not the right age or the circumstances aren't just so, you're on your own.

Bureaucratic red tape makes it damn near impossible for American citizens to receive help.

I applied for Medicaid and Disability.

I was denied Medicaid. I have no idea why.

Disability is another animal altogether. It takes months upon months to get a decision. The majority of the time, Disability is denied the first time around. And the second. And even the third. And sometimes beyond.

Since I have suffered this latest HS flare-up going on nine months at this point, it will be more than a year – maybe even longer – before I am back on my feet. Due to the size of my afflicted area, surgery will be done piecemeal: a small area at a time. Which means several surgeries, several recuperation periods, during none of which I will be able to withstand sitting or standing to perform a job.

What is a person supposed to do? Live on air? Under a bridge? How do these government institutions expect people to survive waiting for them to determine that you need these benefits?

It is frustrating to deal with this sort of mentality.

When these benefits are handed out freely to non-American citizens, it's enough to edge the frustration to fury.

If those benefits can be handed out so freely to refugees, why can't those same benefits be extended to me and others like me, even if only temporarily? Even temporary benefits would help.

And why, oh why, do American citizens band together so eagerly to help a devastated region when there is devastation right here in the United States? Children go to bed hungry. Veterans, who fought for the American way of life that most Americans enjoy, sleep on the streets. The elderly live on Social Security benefits that would land a Senator or Congressman in the poorhouse.

And people suffering debilitating illnesses are invisible, ignored and treated as if they don't matter.

Something isn't quite right about all of that.

I have tried, to no avail, to get media attention for HS as well as for my own plight. But I'm not a celebrity. I'm not an important person. The media isn't going to give me the time of day.

If I did something drastic, it might get me on the six o'clock news. But I'm not wired that way. I've been taught to do the right thing, to follow the rules: it's hard-wired into my brain. I can't do something stupid that would land me in jail, even though in jail I would get the medical treatment I need. And on the taxpayers' dime, to boot.

But I cannot do that in good conscience.

The only choice I have is to keep trying.

And keep hoping there will be some kind
of miracle in the process.

Raising HS Awareness

Educating the public about Hidradenitis Suppurativa is a daunting challenge. Especially these days. Apathy replaced compassion years ago, making it exceptionally difficult to bring attention and awareness to the debilitating effects of HS.

In contemplating ways to raise awareness, I've thought up a few ideas. Mind you, some may seem a little unconventional, possibly even drastic. But if drastic measures must be taken in order to raise awareness, so be it.

Golf Ball Sit-In

I've seen images of HS lumps that are the size of golf balls, some even larger. My own lumps are the size of five golf balls all lumped together. All of them together are actually about the size of a tennis ball.

This first idea is based on the comparison of HS lumps to golf balls. Those lumps are about as hard and unyielding as a golf ball and as painful to sit on as a golf ball. If you've ever sat on a golf ball accidentally, you might agree.

79

First, get some volunteers, preferably people who do not suffer HS but know someone who does. These volunteers take pledges from family and friends based upon how long they can sit on golf balls.

I'm not cruel. Three golf balls taped to the seat of a chair and covered with thick padding. It won't be comfortable, nor will it be nearly as painful as actual HS lumps. But it will give people some idea of what it feels like to sit on those HS lumps.

Pledge money gets donated to HS research or HS Support dot org, or any other HS-related agency, or is divided between two or three.

In addition, I'd suggest getting entertainment: give a local band a break, a magician, guest speakers. A local celebrity maybe, or a doctor knowledgeable about HS to speak. Have reps with booths providing free information about HS and possible treatments. A psychologist to address the emotional aspects of HS effects.

Have food, drink and someone selling balloons.

And get media attention. As much as I hate to say it, the best way of getting the word out is to get it on television. Yes, the Internet is a valuable tool, but television remains the foremost best way to get exposure and raise awareness.

Golf Tournament

In keeping with the golf ball theme, I was also thinking of a golf tournament. And it doesn't have to be serious, either. If a Dean Martin/Jerry Lewis type of team could be found, it would provide wonderful entertainment for a crowd. (Personally, I visualize a Sandra Bullock/Melissa McCarthy duo, in character from the movie *Heat*, sans the cursing). Local celebrities would increase interest as well as get that coveted media attention.

Provide free information about HS for donations. Or perhaps donations for autographs from any local celebrities participating.

Of course, take donations for balloons, soda and food sales.

Donations from spectators go to an HS-related agency or divided between two or three.

A Concert. Or Several Concerts.

Give a local band a break and invite them to perform in an effort to raise HS awareness. Ask them to donate a portion of ticket, CD and merchandise sales to HS research.

Not only does the band get exposure, they also benefit from positive promotion for helping a cause. The cause benefits overall with donations and raising awareness.

Have a Fundraising Picnic or Festival

There's nothing wrong with starting small. Some of the biggest events started as small gatherings.

Have a picnic and invite everyone you know. Have them invite others. Have everyone bring a side dish. One person provides hot dogs and hamburgers to cook out.

Accept donations of any amount. Have guest speakers, including people who actually suffer from HS. Have balloons, games with prizes (they don't have to be expensive prizes), sodas and vendors.

Always provide free information about HS.

The same with a festival. Lots of vendors willing to donate a portion of sales for HS research. Or charge a vending fee or do a combination: small vending fee and a percentage of sales.

Clowns, magicians, guest speakers, musicians, artists: the sky is the limit.

Oh, and, by all means, invite local authors – self-published or otherwise – to participate as vendors or speakers.

Whatever it takes to raise awareness, to get the medical profession to acknowledge the debilitation and severity of HS and to find a cure, that is what must be done.

I'm not the only HS sufferer with ideas about how to raise awareness.

So put on your thinking caps, join with family, friends and other HS sufferers. And let's get busy.

Any Celebrities with HS?

One should not have to be a celebrity in order to get attention.

I am loath to say this, but our country is structured in such a way that celebrities rule the airwaves.

Unless, of course, you commit a crime. Then you're all over the six o'clock news and everybody knows your name. But that's not really the attention we need to focus on Hidradenitis Suppurativa. We're going for compassion and understanding, not incarceration.

However, if a celebrity was struck by HS, the entire world would be aware of it.

As sad as that is, it is true.

Should a celebrity suffer from HS, it would benefit those of us without celebrity status. It would have almost an immediate impact. Doctors would hustle to find the cause and the cure. People would recognize the agony HS sufferers endure. Maybe even the medical profession would show more compassion to those of us with HS.

The next best thing would be a celebrity spokesperson. Preferably one who knows what HS is or knows someone who suffers from the malady.

84

Of course, the only drawback (did I just say only?) is that celebrities expect to be paid. Even when it's for a good cause.

A celebrity spokesperson may be a lovely thought, but, without finances, it's hardly more than a pipe dream.

The bottom line is that raising awareness about HS rests upon the shoulders of those of us down here in the trenches. The women and men actually going through the debilitating pain, the depression, the isolation and the frustration of knowing HS is a lifetime battle. We are the ones responsible for getting the job done.

It is a goal more difficult for us non-celebrities to accomplish based simply on our non-celebrity status. It will require determination, perseverance, patience and tenacity far and above what we are normally capable of.

Most important, it will require solidarity among the greatest number of HS sufferers possible. Numbers cannot be ignored. The combination of a multitude of voices will carry over and above protests and ignorance: We will be heard.

Our requests, no, our *demands* for better treatment, more research and finding a cure cannot be ignored indefinitely. It will take time, but, eventually, researchers, doctors and the public will realize something must be done. We deserve better treatment. We deserve a cure.

We owe it to ourselves to form a united front to accomplish these goals.

We can create our own media attention by combating the ignorance of HS as a group; as a team, if you will. One big team.

Celebrity status may get attention to HS more quickly. But doing it ourselves may be more meaningful.

Long Term Hidradenitis Suppurativa

I don't know the "record" for the longest endurance of a bout of Hidradenitis Suppurativa. I only know I have dealt with it for eight months at this point.

I have watched, literally, as first one golf-ball sized lump after another formed. Unfortunately, they formed on my right thigh and on the outer portion of my labia. I currently have about several golf-ball sized lumps on the thigh and three or four more on the outer labia. The ones on the outer thigh clumped together to form the size of a tennis ball.

How long can a person endure this mess before it becomes septic shock? Or contracts a/an MRSA infection? Or becomes squamous cell carcinoma?

It isn't by choice that I have not had surgery to remove the lumps. You see, in America, if you do not have health insurance and you do not have money, you do not get the treatment you need. It is that simple.

I've been to two different emergency rooms. I was denied treatment by a surgeon due to my inability to pay one of the emergency room bills.

I currently have to go to a local hospital system which treats indigent patients. Or, they are supposed to treat indigent patients. They'll treat you if they feel like it.

With my first two surgeries, I had full time jobs and health insurance at the time. Neither surgeon hesitated to perform the surgery necessary to relieve me of the physical distress caused by HS. THEN, the surgeons addressed other issues of which they were aware prior to the surgery.

Which makes sense. Get rid of what is causing the most stress, the biggest burden, the most pain, and the patient is in a better frame of mind to deal with other things, get back to work, get on with life.

That isn't the way this local hospital system works. They hold the surgery hostage in order to make you jump through their hoops.

The first time, surgery was denied because they wanted me to get my A1C number under control. I get that. Diabetes hinders healing. But can we alleviate my pain so I can get back to work first? I have to support myself.

The second time, surgery was denied. The exact words were, "We're not doing surgery until you quit smoking." An ultimatum.

Sure, I'm aware smoking isn't good for you. I'm aware smoking is "linked" to HS. But there is no irrefutable proof that it is a cause or even a contributor. If it were, then EVERYONE who smoked would suffer HS. Capeesh?

What really boiled me about that is that, once again, surgery was withheld, thereby it was held hostage.

On the third clinic visit, they were ready to put me in the hospital right then and there. Why do they do that? Are they ignorant of the fact that you may need to make some arrangements first?

As it happened, I was being evicted from my home the very next week. I needed to pack. I had no choice but to tell them I couldn't go into the hospital that day.

I thought they had set up surgery for a couple of weeks after that visit. It's a good thing I called. After being transferred four times, I finally discovered I was NOT scheduled for surgery. I was scheduled for a regular clinic visit.

This cut me to the core. Because of the move and quite a few other factors, I didn't have the money to pay for the clinic visit, or pay for someone to take me to the clinic and wait to find out whether or not they were going to admit me for surgery. With this hospital, there are simply no guarantees. Especially as wishy-washy as they had been about doing the surgery.

By the time I return for the clinic visit, it will be nine months – almost to the day – since this latest flare up. Believe me, I recall the very MOMENT this flare up began. But that's another story.

In the meantime, the latest round of antibiotics ran out. Which means the swelling, inflammation, excessive drainage and excruciating pain have returned with a vengeance.

How much longer must I tolerate this? How much longer CAN I tolerate this?

It's disturbing that I must depend upon the callousness of some surgeons at an indigent clinic for my health care. From what I have witnessed of their attitudes, they truly do not care whether I live or die or grow mushrooms in my crack.

I am in constant pain. I am at risk for staph, MRSA infections, septic shock or squamous cell carcinoma. Health care professionals should be aware of these risks for HS.

Get rid of the problem. Address other stuff once those risks have been decreased or taken out of the equation altogether.

I really have no desire to set some kind of world record for longest time spent enduring this crap. Nor do I desire a staph or MRSA infection, septic shock or carcinoma, all of which could create complications and kill me. I want this stuff gone. I want it out of me.

What is so difficult to understand about that?

Feeling the Flare-Up

October 14, 2015. That was the day my latest Hidradenitis Suppurativa flare-up began.

Two weeks prior, the temporary job assignment I was working ended. But the story actually begins back in August.

While at the Decatur Book Festival, I was invited to be a vendor at the Emergency Management conference in Oak Ridge, Tennessee, that upcoming October. The invitation came as a direct result of a sale of *Nero's Fiddle*. I was delighted.

I made hotel arrangements in advance. By the time the job assignment ended, it was too late to cancel. Besides, it was an opportunity to meet people in the field of Emergency Management, a field that prepares for disasters and assists in recovery afterward. Surely, they would be interested in the topic of an electromagnetic pulse attack.

So I forged ahead with my plans. I attended both days of the conference.

I must clarify something here: the older I get, the more nervous I am about driving. I'm not nervous about my driving skills. It's all those other people out there with such little regard for safety or life, whether it is their lives or the lives of others that make me nervous.

Though the drive seemed daunting, I was determined.

I made it there fine, much to my own surprise.

It was the drive back home when I ran into trouble.

At the time, I was already experiencing a small flare-up on the outer side of my labia. Though it was messy and somewhat painful, it wasn't intolerable. You build up a tolerance to pain when you suffer from HS.

I knew the way back home. I had memorized it as well as written it down.

I left the conference around 3:00. The drive was about four hours. I should, hopefully, miss the worst of rush hour traffic.

I stopped to fill up for gas before leaving Oak Ridge. And made the mistake of asking for the quickest route back to the Interstate. I was given directions. And I followed them to the Interstate.

I drove. And drove. And drove. Until I finally realized something wasn't quite right. I hadn't seen any signs directing me to I-75 which would take me back to Atlanta.

I pulled off and made inquiries. The directions I was given were a straight shot:

right into downtown Nashville. Not where I wanted to go.

I was given more directions and I consulted my map. I mapped the route I needed to take: a highway which would eventually lead me around Chattanooga to I-75. A long way out of the way, but the best route from where I was at that moment.

I was in the car and off again.

I stopped about an hour later and filled up again. I calculated from the amount of time I had already driven that this fill up would get me back to Atlanta. Dusk was falling. I didn't want to have to stop again until I pulled up to my door.

I was stressed to the max. Driving at night was worse than driving in general. I was upset with myself for getting off track in the first place and knowing it would soon be dark wasn't helping.

But I trooped on.

During that part of the drive, I began to feel a tingling sensation in my outer right thigh. I knew exactly what it was.

I considered stopping, even for a little while. But I was afraid if I stopped, I just wouldn't get back on the road to go home. Besides, it didn't matter. Taking a rest break would not have delayed nor stopped the impending flare-up. So I kept driving.

In the mountains outside Chattanooga, it was full dark and the roads became quite twisty. But I was lucky. I got behind a semi-truck.

Now, normally, those big rigs make me nervous. But not this driver. S/he drove the speed limit – sometimes below – on those winding roads while cars in the lane beside us drove much too fast.

I ended up staying behind that big rig all the way to the I-285 perimeter around Atlanta as though s/he was a guardian angel (and maybe s/he was), the whole time acutely aware of the growing sensation in my thigh.

Yes, I knew it was a flare-up. Little did I know at the time it would be the worst flare up I have experienced thus far. Little did I know I would have so much difficulty getting treatment. Little did I know the flare-up would quickly reach the point of being debilitating.

Little did I know that going on nine months after that incident, my HS would be so grotesquely out of proportion or so painful or that I would still be trying to figure out a way to get surgery for relief.

It may be a good thing I had no inkling at the time of what lay ahead. Had I known the extent of the debilitation and suffering, well, I may not have made it home that night.

But when you know, when you can tell beyond a shadow of a doubt the moment when an HS flare-up is occurring, that is just way too familiar for comfort.

I have no way of knowing who that driver was and thereby, no way of thanking her or him (ya know, it could very well have been a woman driver). But I hope that all the guardian angels in Heaven protect her or him each time s/he fires up that truck.

Analysis of HS

I'm no doctor or scientist. I may not have a super high IQ, but I am capable of thinking logically.

Currently, research into the causes of Hidradenitis Suppurativa is next to nil. There is no research organization set up for the specific purpose of delving into this vile and inexplicable illness that is quickly becoming an epidemic. Case studies have yet to be conducted and it seems that not many doctors are interested in documenting the effects of HS; something which would prove beneficial for research into the cause and possibly a cure.

The possible causes listed by the medical profession are a joke: obesity, smoking, blah, blah, blah.

I'm not disputing the contributing factors of these things. I question the validity of them because not a single one of those factors pertains to EVERYONE who suffers from HS. Nonsmokers as well as smokers; thin people as well as those who are overweight, etc., etc. If smoking caused HS, ALL smokers would suffer from it. If weight were a factor, all those who were overweight would also suffer.

These results are inconclusive from the fact alone that they are not all-inclusive.

I thought that was the first rule of science: results have to be conclusive. Otherwise, you have to wipe the slate clean and conduct the experiment again.

What really troubles me about those possible causes is that each and every one of them places the responsibility of HS directly in the lap of those suffering from it. Those causes do not pinpoint the precise cause, nor do they offer a solution. Which provides absolutely no comfort or compassion to the HS sufferer.

As I stated, I'm no scientist. But I do recall in science class the importance of finding the common denominator in any scientific experiment in order to extract a conclusion.

Research has not been conducted to discover any such common denominator in HS sufferers.

Granted, symptoms and effects are as varied as the individuals attacked by HS. But it seems to me, logically, there has to be some commonality between them.

Since HS is not contagious – and thank all the heavens above that it isn't – the explanation for why so many people are rapidly falling prey to it lies with the commonality between them.

I have a few thoughts on the matter.

Preservatives

There is not a single item of food on a supermarket shelf which does not contain preservatives. It's a wonder we're not all mummified (zombie apocalypse, anyone?)

Take a look at the expiration dates on the food you buy, particularly canned food items. Some of those dates are two and three years beyond the date they're purchased. How much preservatives are in a can of green beans that makes them still edible two years from now? What preservatives are in that can of green beans?

They may be listed on the label, but I get a feeling maybe not all of them are listed. Even if all of them are listed, some of them are things we don't know or understand.

Those preservatives go into our bodies once they are consumed. What effects do they have on us? Are these preservatives also preserving our innards? Or do those preservatives collect within our bodies and attack at will? Anybody ever studied that?

Unfortunately, preservatives are unavoidable. They're in everything from canned and packaged foods to sodas, coffee and tea.

Genetically Modified Food

Was genetic modification of food conducted during the fifties and sixties?

The idea of messing around with what nature provides burns my cyst-riddled ass. Simply because you are capable of doing something does not give you the right to do something.

And what exactly is in that genetically modified food? Truth be told, no one really knows except for those doing the modifying. But I do know it's the use of chemicals the human body was not meant to ingest.

Fluoride

Yes, we've all grown up using toothpaste. But did you know that fluoride is toxic? It's a poison. Yet every day, every person who brushes his or her teeth ingests this poison. Why on earth it is used in toothpaste is beyond me.

Deodorant

The medical profession claims there is no correlation between underarm deodorant and shaving and HS. I am here to dispute that claim.

I've stated earlier that I got HS lumps in my armpits. I noticed they formed after I shaved so I stopped shaving. I still got them periodically: they were much less frequent when I stopped shaving.

I stopped using underarm deodorant for no other reason than being out of work for a while. That's when the lumps completely stopped forming in my armpits. I completely stopped using underarm deodorant. Thankfully, I haven't had any more lumps appear in either armpit since.

My personal conclusion: there is most definitely a correlation. Further research should be conducted about that.

The exact ingredient in the specific brand needs to be isolated. I used cheap deodorant: whatever was on sale. I simply could never afford the expensive stuff. That is not to say the cheap stuff is more prone to prompt flare-ups. It just means all deodorants need to be researched for their effects on HS.

Things to think about

Is it in the foods we eat? Is it in the chlorine and other chemicals in our water supply? Is it in the soaps we use? The shampoos? The conditioners? The laundry detergents, the fabric softeners, and any of dozens more products that advertising insists we can't live without?

Have we created our own Pandora's Box and unleashed this illness upon ourselves?

HS patients are not to blame if that is the case. The unsuspecting consumer needs things such as food, soap, and laundry detergent for daily life.

The problem is truly not with the fact these things are needed and necessary. The problem is what goes into them that has long-term effects on our bodies.

If any of the above-mentioned items are responsible for HS, what else could they be responsible for? What other illnesses could they contribute to?

It's like the original Batman movie – you know, the one with Michael Keaton and Jack Nicholson – where The Joker puts something into all types of products that makes people break out profusely and die with a smile on their faces.

Except HS sufferers aren't smiling.

And while the inclusion of harmful chemicals may not be intentional, those chemicals could be the very things responsible for a number of illnesses suffered by millions. Including HS.

We are at a crossroads. Though misdiagnoses still occur, more and more people are subjected to the horrible effects of HS every day. And yet, the public and the medical profession alike remain in the dark about this illness. Everything from its very existence to its cause, treatment and a cure remain a mystery.

Normally, I love a good mystery. But this is one that needs to be solved and solved quickly. Before it reaches pandemic proportions.

When Family Doesn't Care

"Go get a job."

I was told those words by my nephew recently. On Facebook, no less. He's a grown man, but obviously not man enough to confront me face to face.

The whole thing started when I posted some items that my mother wanted to sell. One of the items was a bentwood rocker. It needs some refurbishing, she needs the money and the space. I put in the post that the money was for surgery, hoping it would help to sell the rocker.

My nephew hit the roof. He accused me of talking my mother into selling her items.

Truth be told, the rocker and a mirror were the only items that were hers and she is eager to be rid of them. A printer used to belong to my older brother and the television set was mine.

Words were exchanged. I wasn't polite. I didn't care. Still don't.

Then he hit me with "go get a job."

Dealing with Hidradenitis Suppurativa is bad enough. But when you are surrounded by people who offer absolutely no moral support whatsoever, and who, basically, just don't care about you, it makes it all the worse.

104

I am not the only person whose family operates in such a manner. I have read posts and stories by people whose families have told them HS is their own fault. That it's because of their lifestyle or their weight. So I am not alone in this dilemma.

My best friend came to my defense in the exchange. I love her for that.

Someone deleted the entire exchange.

But my friend did what family is SUPPOSED to do: she spoke up on my behalf, defended me, and gave me moral support.

She also offered to move me to Illinois. I'm seriously considering taking her up on the offer. Her family has always shown me moral support. They've helped out financially on occasion. Though I hate to say this about my own family, her family has been more like family to me than my own.

When I can finally have surgery, how can I possibly heal in this atmosphere?

If I could have worked to prevent moving in with my mother, believe me, I would have. I would still be in my apartment. Not grand by any means, but it was mine. There was lots of light. Maybe not a lot of space, but more than there is now. My mother's apartment is half the size of my old one. The room where I reside is barely large enough to accommodate my bed.

And my poor kitty cat has to stay shut up in that one room. My mother's cat would jump on her if they were in the same room together. My cat is 16 years old and I'll not have that cat jumping on her. My baby's been through enough.

I didn't think my self-esteem could sink any lower.

It is sad when families are not families. My family has never been a family. Except by obligation of blood.

I know where my nephew is coming from, in a manner of speaking. He is influenced by another family member who feels this way. This family member and I have never particularly liked each other. My nephew is apparently incapable of thinking for himself and must rely on others to determine and shape his thinking.

He was repeating what he was told by this other family member.

After the exchange on Facebook, I unfriended and unfollowed my nephew.

Five minutes later, my sister-in-law's computer was retrieved. It was the only Internet connection I have. Had. I won't get it back often or soon.

I've been here before. It will get worse as time goes on. The battle for – what? I do not know. Superiority, maybe?

I don't know, but I do know it is a battle that shouldn't be raging. Family shouldn't be like this. But I know my family is not the only one which is this way.

I may have been better off living in my car. But somehow I think my kitty cat would have liked the car even less.

I've lived in Georgia most of my life. I was born here.

But Illinois is looking mighty good right now.

Down the Drain

I cry in the shower.

The act of weeping in front of my mother requires explanation. Ironically, even with an explanation, the conversation turns to how it affects her. It doesn't really matter what I am going through.

This is the price paid for needing a roof over one's head.

There is no relief from the mental and emotional anguish, let alone the physical pain of Hidradenitis Suppurativa. There is nowhere to hide. Staying in my room is out of the question. Even if I fall asleep, there will come a knock on my door to awaken me, if for no other reason than to ask me if I'm being a hermit.

My mother is moody; has always been moody. It doesn't take much to set her off. Most of the time, it's a mystery as to what has set her off. Maybe the milk jug was put in the refrigerator the wrong way. Or the dishes weren't placed in the drain correctly.

The next thing you know, there is the slamming of cabinet doors. Dishes are loudly plopped onto the counter. There is muttering, but who knows what is said?

Ask what's wrong and the slamming gets worse.

Before I moved in, I told my mother how sick I was. I told her that I slept a lot because of the pain. I don't know if she wasn't listening or simply didn't wish to hear.

I think she expected it to be just like it was after my father passed away in 1988. I moved back from California and spent the next 15 years of my life catering to her every whim. I was there the day of her gall bladder attack.

When she had knee replacement surgery, I was working a full time job. There was a full house living there at the time. But I was the one who came home from work, grabbed supper and a change of clothing, then drove to the hospital to sleep in an uncomfortable recliner by her bedside at night.

Fortunately, I belonged to a gym only minutes away from my job. I was up early, went to the gym, worked out and went to work. I did this every day for about a week.

Neither of her sons paid her a visit while she was in the hospital.

My mother was with me for both of my previous surgeries. Her choice, not my insistence or request. A bitchy nurse made some derogatory comments at the second surgery about how my mother shouldn't be going through this.

I've really not had much luck with medical professionals.

But my mother also stayed with me for a while after both surgeries. She knows what I went through.

So why doesn't she understand now?

Ironically, I spent my entire life trying to earn enough money so that I could take care of my mother, as well as myself. Life, however, never met me halfway. I've barely been able to take care of myself financially, much less get enough money together to take care of both of us.

She is 88 years old. I suppose she expects things to be a certain way. And she has a right to. But as much as I would like to cater to her every whim, I cannot at this time.

And I feel her resentment about that. She is angry because I am sick.

And that hurts.

I cry in the shower. My tears go down the drain.

Sick and Tired

When you suffer chronic pain and illness such as HS, you reach a point where you just get sick and tired.

I reached that point several months ago. I've been in a perpetual state of sick and tired for some time now.

I am sick and tired of being told that surgery won't be done, regardless of the reason. No reason is good enough for putting my health at risk.

I am sick and tired of people who simply do not grasp how much pain I am in on a daily basis.

I am sick and tired of being expected to do things which irritate this condition: normal things like going for a drive or driving to the store, carrying heavy bags laden with groceries or even cooking.

I am sick and tired of asking for help only to be told no for various reasons: you don't qualify, you're not old enough, you got a place to live why do you need help?

I am sick and tired of my poor kitty cat being cooped up in one room when she's accustomed to roaming an entire apartment.

I am sick and tired of the itching, which no doctor has addressed nor suggested anything for relief.

I am sick and tired of the excessive drainage; disgusting, nasty drainage that just won't stop.

I am sick and tired of worrying about money, worrying about how I'm going to get more pads, more cat food and more of the few essentials that I need.

I am sick and tired of filling out paperwork, the need for paperwork to prove I have no income, the insistence that paperwork be done or nothing will be done.

I am sick and tired of not being able to comfortably sit in a chair without excruciating pain.

I am sick and tired of being without the Internet.

Being sick and tired is frustrating. And tiring. And unavoidable.

Keeping up a brave and positive front is nigh impossible when you're in a no-win situation. The constant search and mental effort to find solutions only to hit brick wall after brick wall are enough to drain your body of physical energy and the desire to do anything at all.

Keeping hope alive becomes a Herculean feat.

You rest. You sleep. You go at it again. All the while still feeling sick and tired of the bureaucratic nightmare – not to mention the crap HS constantly delivers – that stands between you and being healthy. Or at least feeling better.

I am sick and tired of all this mess. But mostly, I am sick and tired of being sick and tired.

I Don't Need Anger Management

Everybody needs to stop pissing me off.

It may be a meme in jest, but it's true.

I find it ironic that people are not allowed to display anger. Especially these days when there is so much to be angry about.

Granted, anger can be taken too far. Some people take their anger out on others to the point of doing them physical harm. That type of action crosses the border between justified anger and outright rage.

But try and display or voice justified anger at the establishment or the medical profession and you hear labels such as *troubled*, *unpatriotic*, *psychotic* and a number of other derogatory labels that completely miss the point you're trying to make.

It can land you in jail, in the psych ward or in anger management classes.

To make matters worse, the injustice against which you're speaking goes unheard and ignored.

Nothing in this world makes me angrier than to be told I can't have medical treatment or surgery because I am unable to pay or have no health insurance. Or for any other reason.

To voice my anger against this means absolutely nothing. Except to get a little red flag in my medical file labeling me as Heaven knows what. Go ahead and make note of my anguish. At this point, I just don't give a damn.

Because my anger is justified. It is directed at people who ***CHOOSE TO NOT DO THE RIGHT THING.***

We all inherently know right from wrong. Most of us are also taught the difference along the way. NOT doing the right thing is a choice.

For instance, it is NOT right to deny someone medical treatment due to inability to pay or lack of health insurance. It is NOT right to postpone surgery for any reason when a patient is in as much distress as caused by HS.

It is NOT right that the decision for health care rests in the hands of those not affected by the distress of the patient, instead of being in the hands of the patient themselves.

It is NOT right to deny someone Medicaid without a clear cut reason. It is NOT right to force someone to wait such a long period of time before determining if s/he is eligible for Disability. It is even more NOT right to deny Medicaid and Disability to people who obviously need it.

The list of things in this world which are not right is terribly long.

I understand the anguish which pushes some people to perform acts of desperation. The line between middle class and poor gets more blurred each day. People who were once able to make a living find themselves in dire straits and they see no other options.

Anger and desperation mount to the point they attempt robbery or get into fights, both of which can have fatal consequences.

Those same people could use that anger to bring about change instead of placing themselves and others in harm's way. Doing this, of course, takes time and patience. We have been brainwashed into believing in instant gratification: that if we want something now we are entitled to it now. Working towards a goal simply takes too long and too much work to accomplish, regardless of the rewards of working towards that goal.

To say I have not fantasized about stealing money would be a lie. I'm no saint and thinking about doing bad things is part of human nature. But fantasizing is as far as I take it.

I know it is ***NOT THE RIGHT THING TO DO***.

Instead, I channel my anger. I write it out. I work on novels. I plot and plan, establishing an HS Fund to help others in similar situations to my own. It takes time and energy, but I would rather put my anger to productive use rather than lash out and be forced to participate in anger management classes. I couldn't sit for them anyway.

We live in a world where, every day, more people choose not to do the right thing. Fighting the impulse to act on feelings of anger and desperation is as difficult as it is to choose to do the right thing.

Yet there are some people who make that choice with no compunction whatsoever, simply because there are protocols in place which justify the choice. Doctors deny treatment because they are entitled to do so.

When it comes to how we handle those decisions, there are also protocols in place: protocols which rank much higher than hospital or doctor policies or even judicial laws.

Those are the protocols by which we should be living and not the man-made protocols put in place by men in power.

People seem to forget about that. Mankind has established this world in which we live, a world which rotates on a spindle of greed, and not the spindle of goodwill upon which it was originally created.

I may die from HS, a completely unknown author. My books may never sell or I may not live to see them sell. I may not even live to see the HS Fund to fruition.

But when I die, I will die knowing I tried to do the right thing. I didn't allow my anger to become rage. I used my anger to fuel my creativity and my desire to make change.

THAT is real anger management.

Are Bioethics at the Root of HS Treatment Denial?

It's a good thing a strict bioethics system isn't in place: you know, the type of bioethics that believes a person with a chronic illness should be denied treatment until s/he dies.

If that were the case, I would probably be one of the first to go.

I learned about bioethics from reading a Dean Koontz novel. I thought I was reading fiction. I was appalled to learn that bioethics are real. There are people out there who believe treatment should be denied a baby born with health issues so that a healthy baby may live.

There are bioethicists out there who do not condone such mentality. There are others who want to make it policy.

Those evil bioethicists believe it isn't just babies who should be denied treatment. They believe anyone suffering from a chronic illness should be denied medication and treatment until they simply die off. They believe this provides a better quality of life for those people who are healthy. They believe it frees up resources for those healthy people.

119

I have to ask: If those people are healthy, why do they need the resources?

If those inhumane bioethics became policy, it would eliminate people suffering from diabetes, MS, Parkinson's, Gehrig's, disabled people, people suffering with Hidradenitis Suppurativa: basically anyone who didn't live up to the definition and expectations of "healthy." And those definitions and expectations of healthy would be set up by those bioethicists.

The goal of bioethicists who believe in those types of policies is to "weed out" all the unhealthy people in order for healthy people to have a better quality of life. "Survival of the fittest" is their creed.

It makes no sense. How would the elimination of unhealthy people make for a better quality of life for healthy people?

It is frightening to think about. But when I ponder how many people are in a situation similar to my own – unable to work due to a chronic debilitating disease, who are probably denied treatment due to no health insurance and no money – I have to wonder: are those bioethics already in place?

Are bioethicists using the lack of insurance and money to deny less healthy people the treatment they need? Are bioethicists that much in control of who gets treated and who doesn't? Have they managed to infiltrate those positions?

Such a bioethics plan would not be announced. It would be done quietly, in such a way that no one would notice or even question unethical decisions. It is subtle. It creeps in, one decision at a time, like the ghost or monster in those scary movies.

Denying treatment is an unethical decision of gargantuan proportions, regardless of the reasons for the denial or the treatment denied.

Do I believe in conspiracies? In today's world? Are you kidding?

This is all speculation, of course. There is no way to prove whether or not bioethics come into play in the decision to deny treatment. But lack of health insurance and money make plausible – and, of course, *legal* – reasons for the denial. Which would make the implementation of bioethics acceptable without giving patients any legal recourse to reverse the denial of treatment.

The questions I must ask are: How long are we going to tolerate this sort of abuse? How long are we going to allow the medical profession to deny treatment before we get angry enough to fight the system?

What would it take for everyone who has been denied treatment to set aside their differences and stand united to demand we receive the treatment we need and deserve?

Whether intentional or unintentional, subtle or overt, anything is possible. Including the implementation of bioethics policies.

What would it take to overthrow those bioethics policies? Policies which affect every living person on this planet.

It must be soon. Because I have a feeling those policies are moving right along.

Financial Ruin

It has been stated that most people are only one or two paychecks away from living on the street.

Truth is, it's probably closer than that.

I was between jobs when this latest flare-up occurred. It wasn't completely by choice that I had to turn to temp work. I was laid off from a job in 2014 that I had worked for four years. I had planned to stay at that job until book sales improved.

Book sales didn't improve before the layoff.

At the time the flare-up occurred, it wasn't so bad that I couldn't work. It would have been painful, but I could have worked. And I continued looking for another job. Yes, I was collecting unemployment, but I was determined to work. I sent out dozens of resumes each day, made phone calls, sent e-mails.

But employers have ways of finding out your age. During the application process, most of them ask what year you graduated high school. It doesn't take a rocket scientist to do the math.

And we all know employers are geared toward hiring younger people. It's that simple.

123

Unemployment only lasts a certain number of weeks. Once it ends, that's it. You're just outta luck.

Just as the unemployment ran out, I made my first trip to the emergency room. The pain was getting to me and I hoped something would be done about those nasty lumps. I was given antibiotics. Which worked great until they ran out.

Ironically, the only response I got to all those resumes came in February: A data entry position with a government agency, no less. At that point the pain was unbearable: sitting was out of the question.

When I look back, it is amazing I was able to stay in my apartment through the end of May.

I was fortunate that a few friends could help. But everyone has bills to pay; they couldn't continue to help. I am grateful for what they could do.

HS is a parasite, devouring everything in its wake. Including finances.

Pretty soon, emergency room and hospital bills begin to mount. They resemble the leaning Tower of Pisa on your table. There's nothing you can do, but allow them to topple because you definitely don't have the money to pay them or the means to make the money to pay them.

You finally accept the fact that, like most Americans, you will probably die financially destitute and in debt. Your family and friends will have to do a GoFundMe campaign to pay for funeral expenses, as so many people must do these days.

That's not the way I wanted to go. I wanted to go out leaving a legacy behind. Not only the books I write, but enough money from sales to leave to charities.

I don't hold out much hope for that at this moment. A sale of a book or two here and there doesn't yield much. The $1.44 I'm expecting in my account soon isn't going to go far, that's for certain.

I still hope. But that hope is waning.

Time alone will tell.

Counting Down the Seconds

The ticking gets on my nerves.

When we lived in a house, my mother had about three dozen clocks she had collected. She's just crazy about clocks.

That number has been honed down to about one dozen in this matchbox of an apartment.

When it's quiet, the ticking is loud.

I watch the second hand on one of those clocks as it meticulously ticks off the seconds: one more second of my life stolen; one more second of my life filled with pain instead of enjoyment.

It marks off the minutes and hours of my life consumed by Hidradenitis Suppurativa.

The reminder is as annoying as the situation.

I spend every one of those seconds trying to brainstorm some way or another to get the surgery I need.

I have paperwork to fill out for financial assistance at a local hospital. I have to provide all sorts of documentation to accompany this. I find this ironic. First, I have to go to a local library to make copies. I have neither the energy nor the finances to pay for those copies. Furthermore, I then have to get manila envelopes to send in the paperwork. More driving, more money. Lastly, I have to drive to the post office and pay for the paperwork to be sent. You get the picture.

And, no, there is no one who can assist with all of this.

Sure, these things are not expensive. Unless you have absolutely no money with which to accomplish them. Not to mention the pain you must endure to get it done.

The hoops in place to jump through in order to get help are complicated and demanding. While I'm sure they are in place for a reason, individual circumstances should be taken into consideration. Not just for people with HS, but people suffering other debilitating and chronic illnesses such as MS, Parkinson's and even paralysis.

But those people have to jump through the same hoops.

It doesn't seem right.

In the meantime, every second that is ticked off that clock is another second I have not found a solution. It is another second of pain. It is another second of drainage. It is another second I am denied the right to medical treatment.

Seconds add up to minutes to hours to days . . . to months.

And every second I ask the question:
When will this end?

Where Do We Go From Here?

How did the world come to this? How did we reach this point? The point where money means more than anything in this world, including a person's health?

I recall the family doctor we used to see when I was a kid. Dr. Mauldin, a straight shooter if ever there was one. We didn't go to the doctor unless we were truly sick. And we *never* went to the hospital.

But Dr. Mauldin treated you, regardless of your ability to pay. My parents always made sure he was paid for those visits, even if the payment was a month or two later. And he trusted them to make good on the payments.

But I know he had patients who couldn't make good on their payments. Yet he treated them anyway. Because they needed treatment. Dr. Mauldin upheld the Hippocratic Oath, which seems to be moot these days.

How many people die in this world because they cannot pay for medical treatment? And why are they allowed to die?

Why has the medical profession become so callous about people's lives and health?

Why does the system make it so difficult and complicated to get help?

Compassion has gone the way of the dodo bird; it is extinct.

Many, *many* people need help. It seems to me that if the salaries of a few politicians were cut in half, there would be more money in the coffers to help those in need.

Take the movie, *Dave*, for example. Sure, it's fiction. But do you really think there are things in the federal budget that *can't* be cut? Our taxes pay for things we don't even know about and probably wouldn't approve of.

Those decisions are made by politicians with six-figure salaries. Politicians who ride in limousines. And have their own private jets. I'm sure they have other perks of which we, the citizens, have no knowledge.

That money should be rerouted directly into programs to help those in need get medical treatment, food, housing and whatever else is required.

This country was established by our forefathers to escape unfair taxation without representation. We may have representation, but the representation isn't fair at this point. It benefits the rich while veterans sleep on the street, people lose their homes, and those who need it most go without medical treatment and food.

How did we get here?

Where do we go from here? And how do we get there?

HS is No Match for Creative Muse

When my third – and worst – flare-up of Hidradenitis Suppurativa hit, it couldn't have come at a worse time. A temporary assignment just ended and Christmas was coming up. Rent and a host of other bills were due, too.

I don't like being idle. I really don't. I'm all for relaxing as long as I've had a productive day.

HS is counterproductive to any and all goals and accomplishments.

But where there is a will . . .

Writing is my passion. Since the tender age of ten I have pursued the eloquence of the written word.

When this last batch of HS flared up, I realized that sitting in front of my computer was no longer an option. I had to improvise.

The first thing I tried was lying face down on the floor atop a couple of blankets. This is not as comfortable as one might think. Considering the location of my outbreak, it wasn't painful to those, at least not at first. However, it did crush my boobies. And, apparently, something about the blanket didn't agree with them as they broke out in a mild rash, quickly cleared up by a few applications of Neosporin.

I had to try something else.

A dear friend of mine gave me a laptop. I like to tease her about it being the last functioning Gateway laptop on the planet. Mind you, the thing weighs a ton (and a half). It's like picking up one of the eight-inch concrete blocks my father used to work with. It has no Internet connection. It has Word 1997-2003.

But, by gosh, it works. It accomplishes the goal of allowing me to write and save my work. I can then save it to a flash drive and transfer it to my desktop computer, where I once was able to upload my work to the Internet.

The only comfortable position I can find is lying on a sofa or my bed, right leg bent at the knee, left leg extended with most of my weight and pressure on my left butt cheek. Without benefit of pants, as clothing irritates the lumps. Not a pretty picture, but only my cat sees it. As long as she's fed, she doesn't complain.

Even with the pain and the uncomfortable position, characters, ideas and dialogue kept circling in my head. It got to a point I thought I would go stark raving mad between the pain of the HS and these books screaming to be written.

I did the only thing I could do: I fired up the Gateway and started writing.

You must understand something: when I am working on a novel, nothing else exists. Not laundry, not dirty dishes, not a job, and most certainly, not HS. I am aware of the pain on some level. But the turn of the dialogue or the twist of the plot is much too important to allow even one brain cell to acknowledge any stabbing or throbbing pain.

It is one of the advantages of having a creative mind.

As a result, I managed to complete and self-publish three additional titles while under the duress of HS.

This isn't about bragging rights. It's about not allowing HS to control my life. It's about not allowing HS to deny me the one thing which brings me the *most* joy.

I have read other people's HS stories. I admire those who say they will not allow HS to beat them. They maintain their social endeavors and go about their daily lives, thus proving HS will not control how they live.

I admit that my social interaction pretty much came to a halt with this flare-up. My level of mind-over-matter is low on that point. Having the HS in the groin area plays a crucial role in the decision to go outside the door. Regardless of how many pads I use or how much gauze I can squeeze into that crevice, the drainage invariably runs down my leg. It soils clothing and furniture alike.

And, of course, there's the fact that it is painful to sit. It is not possible to have dinner out with friends laying down.

I am aware my stamina in the social battle is limited. But then, I never was a social butterfly. A few close friends are all I need. Those friends are understanding, for the most part, and don't take offense if I turn down an invitation to socialize.

As the HS got progressively worse, I turned down invitations more frequently. Until I've become something of a hermit.

But I crack open the Gateway. And none of that matters. I'm wrapped up in an imaginary world with people who do what I tell them to do (most of the time), and say what I want them to say (well, sometimes they talk back). The world may be passing me by, but I'm creating completely different worlds. Which is exactly what I love to do.

So, no, this isn't about bragging about the number of books I've written. It's about proudly saying that I did something I loved to do, even while I was sick. I didn't allow HS to keep me down so low or so long that I lost sight of the one thing that keeps me going, that brings me comfort and joy, that makes me feel that my day and my time were productive.

If that's what HS wants, if that's what this illness tries to do, well, I think my Creative Muse has a few choice words for it.

I Want to Face My Enemy

When I am finally able to get surgery, I have a special request: I want to face my enemy.

I realize there is little chance that hospital staff will "preserve" the lumps in jars of alcohol for me. They are considered "waste" (as they should be) and probably a Biohazard. Most likely, they will be destroyed in an incinerator (and good riddance to the rubbish.)

So I'm asking that photos be taken of these monsters.

I want to see what I've been battling for nine months now, or however long it will be at the time I can finally have surgery. I want to confront the ugliness that has caused me pain and stress and has kept me in such distress 24/7.

These monstrosities have pervaded my psyche, plummeting me into the deepest, darkest depression I have ever known.

They have taken over my life, preventing me my ability to support myself, interfering with my ability to take care of my precious kitty cat, interrupting my life plans.

These foreign bodies inflicted nonstop pain, forcing me to spend hours with little or no movement and little hope of relief.

Excessive drainage has ruined more of my clothing than I care to think about.

This crap stole my appetite, not only for food, but also for life. The simple pleasure of taking a daily walk was denied me. Visiting with friends became a thing of the past. Just going to the library to check out a book became a distant memory.

There were times, Heaven help me, when HS murdered what little hope I have of ever resuming a semi-healthy life. Forget ever being completely healthy. Without a cure, it is inevitable the damn things will rear their ugly heads again at some point. As long as that is possible, good health is a pipe dream. The most I can hope for is being healthy enough to walk, stand and sit without pain. But I'll sure enough take that and be deliriously happy that I have it.

Because of these vile, despicable things, I was forced to give up my independence, my privacy and what little sanity I possessed.

Being able to see them will assure me they are gone. At least for now.

It will also prove to me – as well as to them – that I am strong enough to withstand. I am stronger than my enemy because I outlasted my enemy. I didn't allow this enemy to overpower me. I didn't fall prey to the hopelessness my enemy tried to inflict upon me.

I did not give up. No matter what this crap threw at me, I did not give up. There were times I wanted to give up, but something inside me, something stronger than these monsters, refused to allow me to give up.

I muddled through. With gritted teeth and clenched fists, I continued fighting. Through the pain, the depression, the life-altering move, the weakness and loss of energy, I kept fighting.

I will be damned if my enemy will take me.

You'd better believe I want to face my enemy. I want to gloat. I have the right to gloat.

If I were allowed to, I'd be there to see the moment when these monsters are destroyed.

Hell, let me light the match.

HS Wish List

I wish Hidradenitis Suppurativa didn't exist.

I wish someone would find or create a cure.

I wish doctors would tell me, "Don't worry about paying right now. Your health is the most important thing."

I wish my friends would stop telling me how strong and tough I am. I wish they understood that I don't feel strong or tough. I feel vulnerable. I feel weak. I feel frustrated and cheated out of my life.

I wish my family would trade their greed for an abundance of unconditional love, compassion, support and understanding. I wish they would acknowledge the pain I'm in. I wish they would stop expecting me to do things for them that cause me pain.

I wish someone would just hold me.

Some days, I wish I were dead. In death, there is no pain, physical, mental or emotional.

I wish I could sleep round the clock.

I wish I could sit in a chair without experiencing excruciating pain that makes me want to scream.

I wish I could go for a walk without pain.

I wish I could work.

I wish my books would sell. One book sale gives me enough hope to last for days.

I wish I could be somebody else, someplace else. Preferably somebody who knows nothing of Hidradenitis Suppurativa and can afford health insurance.

If wishes were riches I'd *be* somebody else someplace else.

I wish good health for anyone reading this. I wish for you to never know the debilitation, humiliation, isolation, depression and pain of Hidradenitis Suppurativa. I wish for you to never take for granted the simple act of painless sitting in a chair, walking or standing.

If you are a healthy individual reading this, I wish I was you.

I Am Not a Hero

It isn't my style to beat my chest with my fists and proclaim hero status. Not when there are others fighting the same fight I'm fighting.

Courage, strength and determination are things I share with every other person battling Hidradenitis Suppurativa. There is no such thing as someone "coming out on top." Every person who survives an HS ordeal or who celebrates remission comes out on top.

A hero is a person who goes far beyond the top. S/he takes her/his own personal suffering and accomplishments outside her/him self. S/he extends her/his personal victory to others also suffering.

Most important, s/he remains humble. No ticker tape parade, no self-proclamation of heroism. Because doing the right thing is not about recognition or acknowledgement. It is about offering a helping hand to those unable to help themselves. It is about doing the right thing.

The label of hero does not apply to me. If any label be used, I prefer it to be the label of . . . inspirational. If my life experiences can serve to inspire others to make something of their lives, or to hold on for just one more day, or to believe that a miracle is possible and on its way, then my life has fulfilled its purpose. Everything I have endured will be worth it.

Though I am a warrior – as are all HS sufferers – a warrior does not a hero make. Speaking up for others does not make a hero. Teaching and encouraging others to speak up for themselves makes a hero.

The true hero in the war on HS will be the person who develops a cure. It will be the person who changes the way the medical profession sees and treats those who cannot afford health insurance or a doctor's office visit. Or it will be the doctor who treats HS patients for the simple reason they need treatment, regardless of rules and policies.

Save the title of hero for those who have truly earned it.

HS Warrior

I am an HS Warrior.

I wield pen and brush and voice as swords and daggers. Words and images are arrows that pierce through my isolation to allow in light where once darkness reigned.

My heartbeat is the drum, calling all to join the fight, knowing victory lies upon the horizon. We need only to see the dawn to exult in our triumph.

Hope is the steed upon which we ride into battle. Determination is my battalion. Courage is our battle cry. None of us knows defeat.

We ride with heads held high, pride resting upon our shoulders. Our strength lies, not only in our numbers, but also in our individuality: That which makes us each unique is also that which sees each of us through the storm of battle.

We survive the pain, the anguish, the desolation thrust upon us. A Warrior knows the challenges. Though the Warrior may be struck down, the true Warrior stands again, ever vigilant in the fight.

Some Warriors will fall. They will be mourned, on and off the battlefield. Their loss will pierce the hearts of kindred Warriors and loved ones alike. Those Warriors remaining will continue the fight in their honor.

Because this is a fight we cannot – *must not* – lose. We will fight until we stand victorious in the brightening rays of the new dawn of freedom: Our freedom from this enemy which shows no mercy and therefore deserves no mercy. We will fight until this enemy is vanquished.

We are stronger than our enemy. Our power lies within our voices, our hearts, our very spirits. That power overpowers all and empowers all of us.

I am an HS Warrior. I am a force to be reckoned with. I will not be defeated by this tyrant, this coward, which dares attack without provocation. I will be the one victorious, wielding my pen, my brush, my voice as weapons against the brutality of such a vile and despicable monster.

I am an HS Warrior.

We are HS Warriors.

In our fight, we are already victorious.

Epilogue

I regret to say this book does not currently have a happy ending.

But it is a hopeful one.

As of the publication of this book, I am awaiting another office visit with the hope I will be admitted to the hospital for surgery. One of many, I was told.

While I am waiting, I am making phone calls and inquiries to see if I can get any assistance at all to help pay for surgery. I'm also making inquiries at a hospital closer to where I live.

And I'm thinking about selling my car. I can no longer pay the insurance. I only drive out of absolute necessity. Once the surgeries begin, I probably won't be able to drive at all. At least that money would pay for food for my kitty cat. Oh, and the pads, underwear and prescriptions that I need.

I'm also planning an HS charity golf game to raise funds to start the HS Fund – USA. This will take time and I'll need lots of help. So I'm attempting to make some contacts, doing my research, getting all my little duckies in a row, so to speak.

And I'm working on a sci-fi time travel series.

All of this in between naps, pain, drainage and family drama trauma.

As you can see, I'm keeping busy. I am determined that HS not take away from me the one thing I love most: writing. And my will to survive this obnoxious illness.

Clearly, I still have a long road ahead of me. But it's a long road behind me, too.

It is still dark in this tunnel. But I wait for the light to shine to guide my way out.

Dealing with HS for going on nine months now doesn't make me a hero, nothing as noble and lofty as that.

But, as one friend tells me, I guess it does make me a "tough old bird."

From the Author/HS Sufferer

Establishing the HS Fund

As of June 20, 2016, the HS Fund – USA is in the planning stage. The "USA" after is to prevent confusion with the HS Fund already established in the UK.

By planning, I mean I'm doing the research to form a nonprofit: the cost to form one, which lawyer would be a good ally and so forth. These things have to start somewhere.

In my mind, the HS Fund – USA will serve two purposes.

The first and foremost purpose is to assist those who have been financially devastated by HS. People who have lost their jobs and/or income, are on the verge of eviction or foreclosure or who cannot get medical help due to no insurance and no money.

In other words, like me in my current situation.

The application process to receive funds will be stringent to ensure that only those people suffering financial stress due to HS are the people who receive the funds. It saddens me to say that, in today's world, there are far too many people who would attempt to get those funds under false pretenses. The strict guidelines in place will be to protect those who truly need the assistance.

I feel it is most important to help HS sufferers first because those who receive assistance will, hopefully, aid in the fight to promote awareness and compassion as well as supporting the goal to find a cure.

The second purpose of the HS Fund – USA is to help support the research to find a cure. There may be grants, which will help in this area. I haven't had the opportunity to research those as of yet. But I will. All in good time.

The HS Fund – USA won't happen overnight. And it certainly won't happen by my efforts alone. I hope to get assistance along the way.

I do not want to do this to make a celebrity out of myself. I want to do this because the feeling of helplessness will always be with me. Being unable to pay bills or rent, being evicted into a no-win situation, having my health held hostage: These painful memories will never leave me. As painful as they are to me, it is equally painful to know that others go through similar experiences because of this horrible illness.

And it simply isn't right. The injustice of it cuts me to the core.

In order to begin establishing the Fund, money is required. Which is why a portion from the sales of ALL my books will be used to begin the process. Enough book sales and more money can be put into the fund.

Money from merchandise sales will also be contributed to the Fund.

Fundraisers are also in the works.

I have to keep my mind busy. Otherwise, I would go mad.

All I ask, dear reader, is that you help spread the word. Every book sale and merchandise sale is more money in the Fund. Every book sale promotes more awareness.

I won't lie to you. Yes, I'll still get something from each book and merchandise sale. Right now, enough to get surgery would send me over the top. Getting surgery and treatment is instrumental to my health and well being which is, in turn, instrumental in establishing the Fund.

Please forgive me if I use part of the sales money to get surgery.

I understand many HS sufferers don't have the funds to purchase books. Believe me, I know. There were, and still are, quite a few books I would love to purchase but I'm currently unable to. I ask those sufferers to encourage family and friends to purchase books.

Tell medical professionals about this one. Some of them could use it.

But with *billions* of potential readers out there and a variety of titles from which to choose with more to come, surely there can be enough sales to take care of everything.

At least, that's my hope.

If anyone is interested in helping to establish the Fund and/or organize fundraisers, please use the contact information in the back of the book to let me know.

Thank you.

Respectfully

Pen

Hidradenitis Suppurativa Websites

As of publication of these essays, there are not many places to find information regarding Hidradenitis Suppurativa. Hopefully, this will improve in the near future.

HS Foundation
www.hs-foundation.org

HS Support
https://hidradenitissuppurativasupportgroup.org/

HS Awareness
http://hidradenitissuppurativaawareness.org/
https://www.facebook.com/hsawarenesspage.1/

Mayo Clinic Overview

http://www.mayoclinic.org/diseases-conditions/hidradenitis-suppurativa/home/ovc-20200012

American Academy of Dermatology
https://www.aad.org/public/diseases/painful-skin-joints/hidradenitis-suppurativa

WebMD
http://www.webmd.com/skin-problems-and-treatments/hidradenitis-suppurativa

National Organization for Rare Disorders

http://rarediseases.org/rare-diseases/hidradenitis-suppurativa/

Decent article online at Dermatology Times, published March 10, 2016

Hidradenitis Suppurativa misunderstood and underdiagnosed

http://dermatologytimes.modernmedicine.com/dermatology-times/news/hidradenitis-suppurativa-misunderstood-and-underdiagnosed

Other Books by Pen

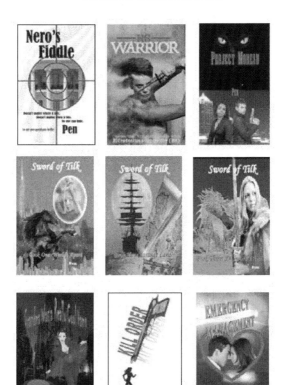

To order these books and others, please visit
www.penspen.wix.com/neros-fiddle

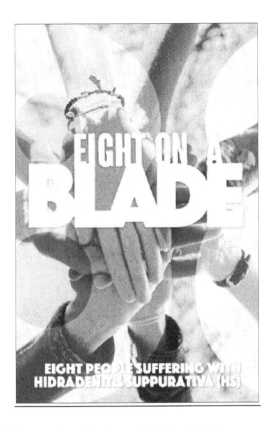

Eight people suffering with Hidradenitis Suppurativa take drastic measures to raise awareness of the virtually unknown affliction.

Their actions provide Zanya Westerly the opportunity to get her foot in the door as a reporter at a local news station.

What follows is sad, enlightening and poignant drama that may result in death.

Visit www.penspen.wix.com/eightonablade

Portions of profits from these book sales are dedicated to establishing the HS Fund – USA to assist those devastated by Hidradenitis Suppurativa.

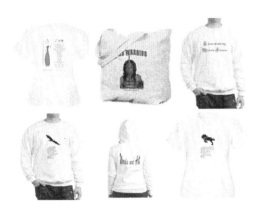

Check out lots more merchandise at
www.cafepress.com/ontheqteez
www.cafepress.com/penspen

Portions of proceeds from all book and merchandise sales will help establish and grow the HS Hope Fund to assist people financially devastated by HS get the medical attention they need. Thank you.

Thank you for reading HS Warrior. If you found the book helpful, please recommend purchasing a copy to family and friends. Also leave a review on Amazon.com.

If you would like to contact Pen, please do so by using the contact form at www.penspen.wix.com/neros-fiddle.

May your life be free from pain and Hidradenitis Suppurativa.

Sincerely,

Pen

65773304R00093

Made in the USA
Charleston, SC
02 January 2017